Immunizations

Guest Editors

MARC ALTSHULER, MD
EDWARD M. BUCHANAN, MD

PRIMARY CARE:
CLINICS IN OFFICE PRACTICE

www.primarycare.theclinics.com

Consulting Editor
JOEL J. HEIDELBAUGH, MD

December 2011 • Volume 38 • Number 4

SAUNDERS an imprint of ELSEVIER, Inc.

W.B. SAUNDERS COMPANY
A Division of Elsevier Inc.

1600 John F. Kennedy Boulevard, Suite 1800 • Philadelphia, PA 19103-2899

http://www.theclinics.com

PRIMARY CARE: CLINICS IN OFFICE PRACTICE Volume 38, Number 4
December 2011 ISSN 0095-4543, ISBN-13: 978-1-4557-7990-1

Editor: Yonah Korngold

Primary Care: Clinics in Office Practice (ISSN: 0095–4543) is published quarterly by Elsevier Inc., 360 Park Avenue South, New York, NY 10010-1710. Months of issue are March, June, September, and December. Periodicals postage paid at New York, NY and additional mailing offices. Subscription prices are $216.00 per year (US individuals), $353.00 (US institutions), $108.00 (US students), $264.00 (Canadian individuals), $415.00 (Canadian institutions), $169.00 (Canadian students), $329.00 (international individuals), $415.00 (international institutions), and $169.00 (international students). Foreign air speed delivery is included in all *Clinics* subscription prices. All prices are subject to change without notice. POSTMASTER: Send address changes to *Primary Care: Clinics in Office Practice*, Elsevier Periodicals Customer Service, 11830 Westline Industrial Drive, St. Louis, MO 63146. Customer Service Health Sciences Division, Subscription Customer Service, 3251 Riverport Lane, Maryland Heights, MO 63043. **Customer Service: 1-800-654-2452 (U.S. and Canada); 314-447-8871 (outside U.S. and Canada). Fax: 314-447-8029. E-mail: journalscustomerservice-usa@elsevier.com (for print support); journalsonlinesupport-usa@elsevier.com (for online support).**

Reprints. For copies of 100 or more, of articles in this publication, please contact the Commercial Reprints Department, Elsevier Inc., 360 Park Avenue South, New York, NY 10010-1710. Tel. (212) 633-3812; Fax: (212) 482-1935; E-mail: reprints@elsevier.com.

Primary Care: Clinics in Office Practice is covered in *MEDLINE/PubMed (Index Medicus) and EMBASE/Excerpta Medica, Current Contents/Clinical Medicine, and ISI/BIOMED.*

Printed and bound by CPI Group (UK) Ltd, Croydon, CR0 4YY

Transferred to Digital Print 2011

Contributors

CONSULTING EDITOR

JOEL J. HEIDELBAUGH, MD
Clinical Assistant Professor and Clerkship Director, Department of Family Medicine; Clinical Assistant Professor, Department of Urology, University of Michigan Medical School, Ann Arbor, Michigan

GUEST EDITORS

MARC ALTSHULER, MD
Department of Family and Community Medicine, Thomas Jefferson University, Philadelphia, Pennsylvania

EDWARD M. BUCHANAN, MD
Department of Family and Community Medicine, Thomas Jefferson University, Philadelphia, Pennsylvania

AUTHORS

MARC ALTSHULER, MD
Department of Family and Community Medicine, Thomas Jefferson University, Philadelphia, Pennsylvania

JOSHUA H. BARASH, MD
Department of Family and Community Medicine, Thomas Jefferson University, Philadelphia, Pennsylvania

EDWARD M. BUCHANAN, MD
Department of Family and Community Medicine, Thomas Jefferson University, Philadelphia, Pennsylvania

ARTHUR L. CAPLAN, PhD
Sidney D. Caplan Professor of Bioethics, Director, Department of Medical Ethics, Center for Bioethics, University of Pennsylvania, Philadelphia, Pennsylvania

CHRISTOPHER V. CHAMBERS, MD
Professor and Director, Clinical Trials, Department of Family and Community Medicine, Jefferson Medical College, Thomas Jefferson University, Philadelphia, Pennsylvania

KATHRYN M. CONNIFF, MD
Assistant Professor, Department of Family Medicine, University of Maryland School of Medicine, Baltimore, Maryland

GARY A. EMMETT, MD
Professor, Department of Pediatrics, Thomas Jefferson University, Philadelphia, Pennsylvania

CHRISTINA M. HILLSON, MD
Department of Family and Community Medicine, Thomas Jefferson University, Philadelphia, Pennsylvania

SANFORD R. KIMMEL, MD
Professor of Family Medicine, Department of Family Medicine, University of Toledo College of Medicine, Toledo, Ohio

DONALD B. MIDDLETON, MD
Professor, Department of Family Medicine, University of Pittsburgh School of Medicine, Pittsburgh, Pennsylvania

GIANG T. NGUYEN, MD, MPH, MSCE
Department of Family Medicine and Community Health, University of Pennsylvania, Philadelphia, Pennsylvania

CHRISTOPHER P. RAAB, MD, FAAP
Clinical Instructor in Pediatrics, Thomas Jefferson University, Philadelphia, Pennsylvania; Pediatrician, Divisions of Diagnostic Referral and Solid Organ Transplant, Nemours/A.I. duPont Hospital for Children, Wilmington, Delaware

MELISSA SCHNEIDER, MD, MSPH
Pediatric Resident, Grand Rapids Medical Education Partners, Helen DeVos Children's Hospital, Michigan

JASON L. SCHWARTZ, MBE, AM
Associate Fellow, Center for Bioethics, Doctoral Candidate, Department of History and Sociology of Science, University of Pennsylvania, Philadelphia, Pennsylvania

SUZANNE MOORE SHEPHERD, MD, MS, DTM&H, FAAEM
Professor of Emergency Medicine, Education Officer, Medical Director of the Fast Track, and Director of Education & Research, PENN Travel Medicine, Department of Emergency Medicine, Hospital of the University of Pennsylvania, Philadelphia, Pennsylvania

WILLIAM HUDSON SHOFF, MD, DTM&H, FACEP
Associate Professor of Emergency Medicine, Medical Director, PENN Travel Medicine, Department of Emergency Medicine, Hospital of the University of Pennsylvania, Philadelphia, Pennsylvania

KATHRYN P. TRAYES, MD
Assistant Dean of Student Affairs and Career Counseling, Instructor, Department of Family and Community Medicine, Thomas Jefferson University Hospital, Jefferson Medical College of Thomas Jefferson University, Philadelphia, Pennsylvania

JUDITH A. TROY
Research Assistant IV, Department of Family Medicine, University of Pittsburgh School of Medicine, Pittsburgh, Pennsylvania

KENDRA VINER, PhD, MPH
Philadelphia Department of Public Health, Philadelphia, Pennsylvania

DANIEL WALMSLEY, DO, FAAP
Clinical Assistant Professor of Pediatrics, Division of General Pediatrics, Thomas Jefferson University/Nemours Pediatrics, Philadelphia, Pennsylvania

BARBARA WATSON, MBChB, FRCP[UK]
Adjunct Associate Professor of Pediatrics, Thomas Jefferson Medical School, Philadelphia, Pennsylvania; Retired from Philadelphia Department of Public Health, Wareham, Massachusetts

ROBERT M. WOLFE, MD
Clinical Associate Professor, Department of Family Medicine, Pritzker School of Medicine, University of Chicago and NorthShore University HealthSystem, Lincolnwood, Illinois

RICHARD K. ZIMMERMAN, MD, MPH
Professor, Department of Family Medicine, University of Pittsburgh School of Medicine, Pittsburgh, Pennsylvania

Contents

Foreword: Immunizations as the Nucleus of Prevention **xi**

Joel J. Heidelbaugh

Preface **xiii**

Marc Altshuler and Edward M. Buchanan

How the Immune Response to Vaccines is Created, Maintained and Measured: Addressing Patient Questions About Vaccination **581**

Barbara Watson and Kendra Viner

This article gives an overview of the immune response to vaccines, including ways in which it is measured and/or augmented to enhance its effectiveness. A brief description is given of the immune response, adaptive immunity, immunologic memory, antibodies, and adjuvants. Given that many young parents and physicians have never witnessed the ravages of vaccine-preventable diseases, it is hoped this article will aid the many people involved in the prevention of infectious disease to understand better the concepts and practicalities of immunization and vaccine development.

Routine Pediatric Immunization, Special Cases in Pediatrics: Prematurity, Chronic Disease, Congenital Heart Disease: Recent Advancements/Changes in Pediatric Vaccines **595**

Daniel Walmsley

Vaccination is a powerful and dynamic weapon in reducing the impact of infectious diseases in children. The field and schedules are constantly evolving, with significant changes resulting in new and exciting vaccines almost yearly. Special cases in pediatrics represent unique challenges and differences in vaccinations. Health care providers need to be knowledgable about the current vaccines and to remain up to date with the constant evolution, as well as be aware of the latest recommendations, warnings, and news about vaccines and their use. This article updates and discusses current but ever-changing routine pediatric vaccination programs.

Adult Vaccination **611**

Christina M. Hillson, Joshua H. Barash, and Edward M. Buchanan

Immunization has effectively decreased the burden of disease on society. Nevertheless, over 50,000 deaths occur annually in the United States from vaccine-preventable disease, and nearly all of these occur in adults. It is essential for primary care physicians to be knowledgeable about the unique immunization-related needs of adults and to be aware of the factors that determine the need for vaccination.

Vaccine-Preventable Diseases and Foreign-Born Populations **633**

Giang T. Nguyen and Marc Altshuler

According to the most recent census data, foreign-born individuals account for more than 12% of the US population. Because many vaccine-preventable outbreaks in the United States have been correlated with disease importation, Congress has mandated vaccinations for numerous immigrant populations. It is essential for primary care physicians to be knowledgeable about the unique immunization-related needs of foreign-born individuals to recognize some of the cultural and linguistic challenges that immigrants have accessing health care and to remember to use each medical encounter as an opportunity to provide necessary vaccinations.

Immunization in Travel Medicine 643

Suzanne Moore Shepherd and William Hudson Shoff

The specialty of travel medicine encompasses a broad and dynamic practice. A thorough pretravel consultation provides an individual with a comprehensive, evidence-based, contextual discussion of the risk profile for specific itinerary-based, travel-related illness and injury, allowing the traveler to use this information in conjunction with his or her personal health belief model, risk tolerance, and experience to decide on an informed management plan. This article focuses on the pretravel consultation with emphasis on the contribution of immunization to traveler's health.

Passive Immunization 681

Christopher P. Raab

Passive immunization employs preformed antibodies provided to an individual that can prevent or treat infectious diseases. There are several situations in which passive immunization can be used: for persons with congenital or acquired immunodeficiency, prophylactic administration when there is a likelihood of exposure to a particular infection, or treatment of a disease state already acquired by the individual. Passive immunization is limited by short duration (typically weeks to months), variable response, and adverse reactions. This article focuses on specific immunoglobulins for preventing or treating infectious diseases, as these are the most likely scenarios one might encounter in primary care practice.

The Course and Management of the 2009 H1N1 Pandemic Influenza 693

Sanford R. Kimmel

The 2009 influenza A (H1N1) pandemic provided a major test to the public health system in the United States and abroad. Although the virus was rapidly identified, it took longer than expected to bring an effective vaccine to market. During the interim the virus demonstrated a predilection for infecting younger persons, particularly those with medical conditions such as asthma or pregnancy, placing them at risk. Early treatment with neuraminidase inhibitors was found to be of some benefit. When the 2009 H1N1 influenza A vaccine became available, there were distribution issues in matching the number of doses to areas of need.

Cancer Vaccines 703

Christopher V. Chambers

The term cancer vaccines encompasses 2 different types of vaccines. Prophylactic vaccines block infection by viruses that can alter host DNA and result in cancer. The hepatitis B vaccine and the human papillomavirus vaccines are examples of prophylactic vaccines that can prevent cancer from developing. More recently, therapeutic vaccines have been developed and used as adjunctive therapy in patients who have already been diagnosed with cancer. Therapeutic vaccines stimulate the host's immune system to recognize cancer cells as foreign and to attack them. Most of the therapeutic vaccines being studied are used in combination with other forms of cancer therapy.

Vaccination Refusal: Ethics, Individual Rights, and the Common Good **717**

Jason L. Schwartz and Arthur L. Caplan

Among the obstacles to the success of vaccination programs is the apparent recent increase in hesitancy and outright resistance to the recommended vaccination schedule by some parents and patients. This article reviews the spectrum of patient or parental attitudes that may be described as vaccine refusal, explores related ethical considerations in the context of the doctor-patient relationship and public health, and evaluates the possible responses of physicians when encountering resistance to vaccination recommendations. Health care providers should view individuals hesitant about or opposed to vaccines not as frustrations or threats to public health, but as opportunities to educate and inform.

Office Immunization **729**

Gary A. Emmett and Melissa Schneider

Nothing has improved disease control as thoroughly as immunizations. In well-immunized populations, there is no flaccid paralysis (polio), almost no epiglottitis or postmeningitis deafness (*Haemophilus influenzae*), and little postviral male sterility (mumps). Immunizations are not perfect; they may cause side effects, some of which have led to the discontinuation of the vaccine when side effects have outweighed the vaccine's protective effects. However, immunization works best not by the protection it provides the individual but by the protection provided to the population at risk. This article discusses the currently available vaccines along with recommendations for their use.

Keeping Up-to-Date with Immunization Practices **747**

Donald B. Middleton, Richard K. Zimmerman, Judith A. Troy, and Robert M. Wolfe

This article presents sources of information for those in practice, administration, or education to stay up-to-date in vaccine recommendations. Web-based repositories predominate in the provision of information. Other sources include newsletters, conferences, journals, expert opinion, community organizations, and books. The promise of the electronic health record remains unfulfilled but improving.

Q & A: Patient to Physician FAQs: Answers to Common Patient Questions About Vaccinations **763**

Kathryn P. Trayes and Kathryn M. Conniff

This article outlines common questions about vaccinations that patients ask their physicians and provides answers to those questions.

Index **777**

FORTHCOMING ISSUE

March 2012
Prenatal Care
David R. Harnisch, MD,
Guest Editor

RECENT ISSUES

September 2011
Gastroenterology
James Winger, MD, and
Aaron Michelfelder, MD,
Guest Editors

June 2011
Palliative Care
Serife Eti, MD, *Guest Editor*

March 2011
Substance Abuse in Office-Based Practice
Robert Mallin, MD,
Guest Editor

Foreword

Immunizations as the Nucleus of Prevention

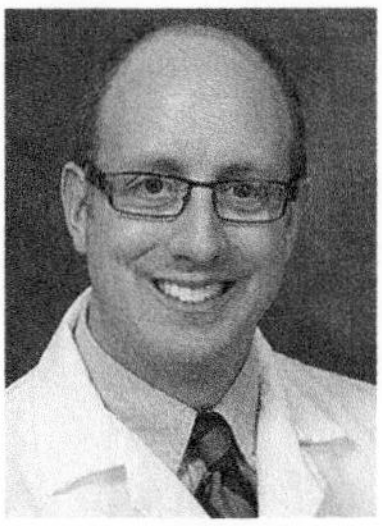

Joel J. Heidelbaugh, MD
Consulting Editor

Every year, I dread flying to conferences for fear of contracting the latest H?N& influenza strain. I also struggle with memorizing the subtle changes in the immunization schedule recommended by the Advisory Committee on Immunization Practices. Like many clinicians, each time I see a child in my practice, the first part of the medical record I review is the immunization registry with the intent of capturing and correcting any missing vaccinations.

Most of us can't begin to understand the potential ramifications of a widespread pandemic, because we haven't lived through one and have only read about outbreaks of deadly communicable diseases in books or heard about them through a distant family member. I contracted chicken pox when I was in kindergarten at age 5 and convalesced at home; then I couldn't return to school because nearly the entire class was infected and school was canceled! When I was a freshman at Siena College in 1989, we had an outbreak of measles that afflicted 45 students. Regardless of immunization status, every student had to receive an additional MMR booster and present a verified ticket prior to attending classes. The threat of national widespread disease and panic originating in the small hamlet of Loudonville, New York became a real possibility. The preface of this volume outlines pre- and postvaccine data that offer great reassurance that when clinicians follow immunization protocols appropriately, such a risk can be greatly minimized.

Recommending immunizations in my current practice assumes two disparate scenarios: the immediate sell and the immediate decline. Most parents agree without hesitation to administer the recommended immunizations to their children. There are, and always will be, parents who feel that such immunizations are not required, are risky (eg, cause autism), and that the threat of sporadic or widespread epidemics of communicable diseases simply won't apply to their offspring. Adults are often more dismissive, especially with regard to getting their yearly influenza immunization. The excuses,

Prim Care Clin Office Pract 38 (2011) xi–xii
doi:10.1016/j.pop.2011.08.001 **primarycare.theclinics.com**
0095-4543/11/$ – see front matter

"my friend got it and he got the flu" and "I've never gotten the flu shot, and I've never gotten the flu, so I won't need it," can be very tough to counter.

Drs Altshuler and Buchanan should be heralded for compiling a unique, practical, and detailed *Primary Care: Clinics in Office Practice* volume dedicated to teaching us not only the importance of the wide array of immunizations, but the science behind what it takes to prevent an epidemic. It is my hope that clinicians who utilize this volume in their daily practices will be suitably equipped with a fantastic resource to portend immunizations as the true nucleus of disease prevention.

Joel J. Heidelbaugh, MD
Ypsilanti Health Center
200 Arnet Street, Suite 200
Ypsilanti, MI 48198, USA

E-mail address:
jheidel@umich.edu

Preface

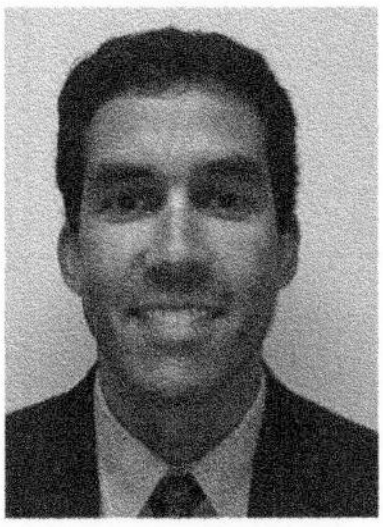
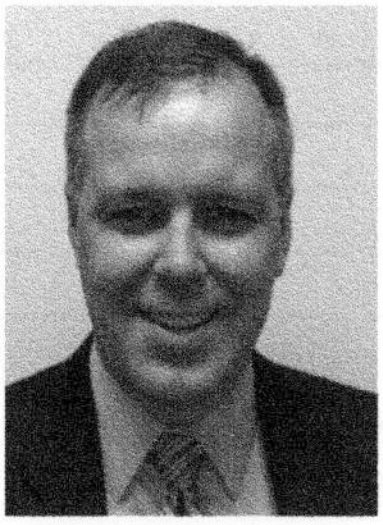

Marc Altshuler, MD   Edward M. Buchanan, MD
Guest Editors

Vaccine science has been a critical field in the control of numerous diseases with infectious and noninfectious etiologies. Through widespread vaccination programs, smallpox has been eradicated globally, while polio has been eliminated from the Western hemisphere and is poised for global elimination as well. One by one, a number of devastating diseases, that in the past were leading causes of worldwide mortality, have been so successfully controlled that most present-day individuals, laypersons, and clinicians alike have no experience with them (**Table 1**).

This success, however, has brought new challenges to the primary care provider. Clinicians must constantly remain updated on the increasing number of available vaccines and their indications. Likewise, they must be alert to the vaccination needs of their patients, who may present to the office with a very different agenda altogether. In many cases, they may be faced with the reluctance or hostility of patients toward vaccines based on fears magnified by the media and Internet.

Unfortunately, even with the universally accepted recognition of the benefits of vaccine administration, many individuals in the United States remain undervaccinated. Statewide initiatives and school-based requirements have increased the numbers of vaccinated children in this country, but the numbers of adults who lack the appropriate vaccinations is astounding. The primary care provider plays an essential role in educating these individuals and bridging the gaps between the undervaccinated and the immunized population.

In this edition of *Primary Care: Clinics in Office Practice*, we aim to educate primary care clinicians to the variety of challenges posed by vaccine science through its implementation in primacy care practice. We begin with an article reviewing the immune response and how vaccines induce immunity. Several articles will then review routine pediatric and adult vaccination, including special populations such as pregnant women, premature babies, and the immunocompromised individual. Proper vaccine administration is also addressed. The next several articles discuss more unique situations of vaccination, including the use of vaccine in foreign-born individuals, travel medicine, pandemic illness, and the importance of immunoglobulins. As mentioned earlier, there still exist may widely held beliefs and concerns that often lead to vaccine refusal; one article addresses the ethics of vaccine refusal. The last few articles bring

Prim Care Clin Office Pract 38 (2011) xiii–xiv
doi:10.1016/j.pop.2011.08.002   primarycare.theclinics.com

Table 1
Present day impact of vaccines compared to the prevaccine era[1,2]

Disease	Prevaccine	US Data 2009
Smallpox	29,005	0
Diphtheria	21,053	0
Pertussis	200,752	16,858
Tetanus	580	18
Polio	16,316	1
Measles	530,217	71
Mumps	162,344	1,991
Varicella	4,085,120	20,480
Hepatitis B	66,232	3,405
Invasive HIB	20,000	3,022

important closure, as we carefully examine the role of clinical trials and the future of vaccine development. We end with two important articles on keeping up to date with current US vaccine guidelines and a Question and Answer section for the primary care provider.

As editors, we wish to thank many individuals who have contributed to this issue. First, we would like to express our highest level of gratitude to the many authors who helped create this important component to the *Primary Care Clinics* series. We recognize their busy lives and appreciate the time and dedication they put into writing their individual articles. Next, we would like to thank our mentor, Chair, and past editor of *Primary Care Clinics*, Dr Richard Wender, who met with us throughout the process, providing us with continued guidance and leadership. And finally, our most sincere thanks to our editors, Yonah Korngold and Joel Heidelbaugh, for their ongoing support and assistance, in addition to the staff at Elsevier, who patiently work with us to create what we hope to be another successful series for *Primary Care Clinics.*

Marc Altshuler, MD
Edward M. Buchanan, MD

Department of Family and Community Medicine
Thomas Jefferson University
833 Chestnut Street, Suite 301
Philadelphia, PA 19107, USA

E-mail addresses:
marc.altshuler@jefferson.edu (M. Altshuler)
edward.buchanan@jefferson.edu (E.M. Buchanan)

REFERENCES

1. Roush SW, Murphy TV. The Vaccine-Preventable Disease Table Working Group. Historical comparisons of morbidity and mortality for vaccine-preventable diseases in the U.S. JAMA 2007;298(18):2155–6.
2. CDC. Summary of notifiable diseases—United States, 2009. MMWR 2011;58(53): 1–100.

How the Immune Response to Vaccines is Created, Maintained and Measured: Addressing Patient Questions About Vaccination

Barbara Watson, MBChB, FRCP[UK][a,b,*], Kendra Viner, PhD, MPH[c]

KEYWORDS

• Immune response • Vaccination • Adjuvants • Antibody titers

The health and life span of the average person living in the United States improved dramatically during the twentieth century.[1] Much of this improvement is a result of advances in public health, including improved sanitation and hygiene, safer and healthier foods, motor-vehicle safety, family planning, and the prevention of infectious diseases through vaccination. The concept of vaccination originated from historical observations dating as far back as 400 BC that individuals who survived a disease rarely got the same disease a second time.[1–4] In 1796, Edward Jenner theorized that milkmaids were often spared from smallpox outbreaks because of prior infection with cowpox.[1] Jenner's theory predated the "germ theory" put forth by Louis Pasteur and Robert Koch that many diseases are caused by microorganisms. These scientists gave us the current definition of a vaccine as a "suspension of live (usually attenuated) or inactivated microorganisms (eg, bacteria or viruses) or fractions thereof administered to induce immunity and prevent infectious disease" (**Table 1**). In subsequent years, effective vaccines would be developed against many devastating illnesses,

[a] Thomas Jefferson Medical School, Philadelphia, PA, USA
[b] Philadelphia Department of Public Health, 6 Sea Street, Wareham, MA 02571, USA
[c] Philadelphia Department of Public Health, 500 South Broad Street, Philadelphia, PA 19143, USA
* Corresponding author. Philadelphia Department of Public Health, 6 Sea Street, Wareham, MA 02571.
E-mail address: Doonholm@gmail.com

Prim Care Clin Office Pract 38 (2011) 581–593
doi:10.1016/j.pop.2011.07.001 primarycare.theclinics.com

Table 1
Vaccine classification

	Live Attenuated	Inactivated
Mechanism of action	• Need to replicate • Existing antibody may interfere • Immunity similar to natural disease—requires T-cell responses, 1 dose protects most, but 2 doses achieve impact on public health and longer memory (CMI)	• No replication • Minimal interference from antibody. Not as effective as live vaccines • Needs 3–5 doses • Immune response is predominantly humoral (ie, antibody) • Antibody wanes with age or time • Booster doses are required • Poorly immunogenic—needs an adjuvant

	Live Attenuated		Inactivated					
					Fractional			
					Protein-Based		Polysaccharide Based	
Vaccine Subtype	**Viral**	**Bacterial**	**Whole Viral**	**Whole Bacterial**	**Toxoid**	**Subunit**	**Pure**	**Conjugate**
Examples	Measles Mumps Rubella Varicella Oral polio Rotavirus LAIV Yellow fever Smallpox	BCG Oral typhoid	IPV HAV Rabies Influenza	Pertussis Typhoid Cholera Plague	Diphtheria Tetanus	HBV Acellular Pertussis Lyme Flu HPV	Pneumo Meningo S.Typhi	HiB Pneumo

Abbreviations: CMI, cell-mediated immunity; HAV, hepatitis A virus; HBV, hepatitis B virus; HiB, *Haemophilus influenzae* type b; HPV, human papillomavirus; IPV, inactivated poliovirus vaccine; LAIV, live attenuated influenza vaccine; Meningo, meningococcus; Pneumo, pneumonia; S.Typhi, *Salmonella typhimurium*.

including diphtheria, measles, meningitis, tetanus, yellow fever, pertussis, and polio. Indeed, the worldwide eradication of smallpox can be attributed to a successful vaccine in combination with a massive global immunization campaign.[1]

Vaccine development is not always consistent and straightforward, however. In part, this is because science has yet to fully understand the immune system and the different responses it must mount to cope with a wide array of distinct pathogens. To ask that a vaccine induce strong and lasting immunity to an infectious agent without itself causing disease is often a tall order. In addition, pathogens themselves are not always stable targets and can evolve ways to subvert the immune response. Two of the world's most insidious microbes, Plasmodium (the malaria parasite) and HIV, have circumvented eradication efforts in this way.[1] Given the complexity of the host-pathogen relationship it is worthwhile to provide a brief overview of the immune response before delving into vaccinology.

AN OVERVIEW OF THE IMMUNE RESPONSE

The central function of the immune system is to protect the host from potentially harmful substances. These substances include living organisms, such as viruses, bacteria and protozoa, as well as nonliving materials such as toxins, drugs, and foreign particles. Once the physical barriers of an individual, which include the skin, mucosal lining of the gut, and air passages, have become compromised, the immune response is activated.[1,5] As the immune system protects its host from invaders, however, it must also be selective, recognizing and ignoring commensal bacteria, environmental antigens and, most importantly, the host tissue itself. Memory, the ability of the immune response to imprint and recall the features of a pathogen so that on subsequent exposures the response is both faster and more robust, is an essential component of both an effective immune response and the development of a functional vaccine.[2,4,5]

Innate Immunity

When pathogens are successful at penetrating the physical barriers of the body, it is the innate arm of the immune response that represents the next line of defense. Macrophages, neutrophils, basophils, natural killer cells, and dendritic cells (DCs) comprise the innate immune system (**Fig. 1**). These cell types release a variety of inflammatory mediators upon recognition of pathogen-associated pattern recognition receptors (PRRs), molecular structures found on microbial surfaces.[6,7] Although PRRs lack the exquisite specificity of the T-cell and B-cell antigen receptors of adaptive immunity, they do allow detection of a wide range of potential pathogens by a small number of receptor genes that are under constant evolutionary pressure.

Innate immunity, though critical, is primitive and nonspecific, paralleling the defense mechanisms used by lower vertebrates. One of its most important properties is the processing and presentation of foreign exogenous antigen in the context of major histocompatibility complex (MHC) class II molecules on macrophages and DCs The most effective antigen-presenting cells (APCs) are DCs, esteemed for their ability to migrate from inflamed tissues to secondary lymphoid organs where they activate naïve T cells and jump-start the adaptive arm of the immune response.[8] Also important for the initiation of adaptive immunity are peptides found in the context of MHC class I. These molecules are located on both APCs and non-APCs, and are responsible for presenting "endogenous" antigens such as those arising from intracellular pathogens like viruses and bacteria, or from tumor proteins.[9]

	Cell Type	Primary Function
Innate Immune Cells	Antigen Presenting Cells: - Macrophages 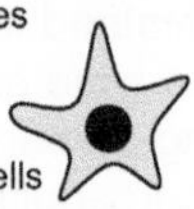 - Dendritic Cells 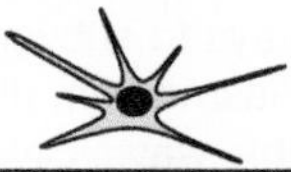	• Engulf and destroy extracellular pathogens and necrotic cellular debris • Present antigen to T cells and induce adaptive immunity
	Neutrophils 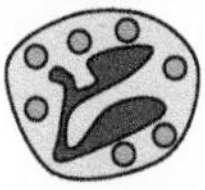	• First-responders to a site of inflammation • Engulf and destroy extracellular pathogens • Release soluble anti-microbial agents
	Basophils 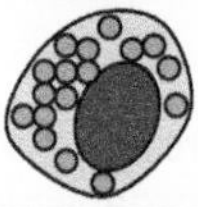	• Release histamine to promote blood flow to tissues • Release heparin to delay blood clotting • Mediate responses to parasitic infection
	Natural Killer cells 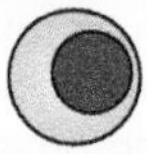	• Lyse infected cells and tumor cells through the release of perforins and granzymes
Adaptive Immune cells	T cells 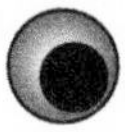	CD4+ T helper (Th) cells • Assist in B cell maturation • Activate CD8+ T cells, macrophages, and DCs • Secrete a wide range a cytokines CD8+ cytotoxic T cells • Lyse infected cells and tumor cells
	B cells 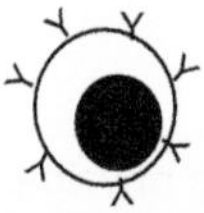	• Produce and secrete antibodies, which help destroy microbes by binding to them and making them better targets for macrophages and DCs.

Fig. 1. Cell types of the innate and adaptive immune system.

Adaptive Immunity

The adaptive arm of the immune response sweeps in behind innate immunity and elicits a response that is specific for the infectious agent. B-cell–derived antibodies and T cells are the primary players in adaptive immunity, and each has evolved to perform distinct functions.[6] Whereas T cells work to destroy infected cells, antibodies are produced to deal with the microbe itself (ie, free virus particles, bacteria, and parasites) (see **Fig. 1**).[9]

T cells

Prior to activation, naïve T cells circulate from the blood through the secondary lymphoid organs, specifically the paracortex of the lymph nodes and the periarteriolar lymphoid sheath (PALS) of the spleen.[9] Restriction to these organs occurs because the T-cell adhesion molecules are highly expressed in these areas.[10] T-cell activation occurs following T-cell receptor (TCR) recognition of peptide-MHC complexes on infected cells. Expression of CD4 or CD8 coreceptors by the T cell aids in the mediation of different types of immune responses. CD8+ T cells recognize peptide-MHC class I complex, and are thus primarily required for defense against microbes that invade and directly release products into the cytosol of cells.[11] Once activated, CD8+ T cells have a wide range of effector functions, including the ability to lyse target cells and recruit other inflammatory cells to the site of infection.[12] CD4+ T cells, by contrast, recognize peptide-MHC class II complexes and compose an important line of defense against intracellular pathogens that are maintained within phagocytic vacuoles of the host cell as well as extracellular organisms, which secrete soluble factors that may be taken up and presented by APCs.[13]

Newly activated antigen-specific T cells produce the proinflammatory cytokine, interleukin (IL)-2, which promotes clonal expansion. Depending on the type of cytokine stimulation given by the infected APC, T cells will further differentiate into 1 of 4 phenotypes, T helper 1 (Th1), Th2, Th17, or Treg, each with its own function in further activating or regulating the immune response.[14] Once an activated T-cell population has effectively contained the infection, it is eliminated by either activation-induced cell death or withdrawal of IL-2 and other growth factors.[15] Although this results in a massive contraction of the activated T-cell population, a small fraction survives as memory cells.[16]

B cells and antibody

B cells develop from hematopoietic stem cells in the bone marrow. Naïve B cells expressing surface immunoglobulin (Ig)M antibody must first survive negative selection, or the deletion of potentially autoreactive B-cell clones, then exit the marrow and migrate to the spleen to undergo further maturation.[17] Most then continue to circulate through the lymphatic system until they encounter foreign antigen. At this point they must receive additional signals from Th lymphocytes to proliferate as plasma cells and undergo immunoglobulin class switching, the mechanism by which a B-cell antibody isotype switches from IgM to IgG, IgA, IgE, or IgD and is produced as a free molecule.[18] Antibodies that have switched classes will recognize the same antigen, but hone to different locations and interact in discrepant ways with immune effector molecules (**Table 2**).

Like T cells, B cells also differentiate into specialized subsets, a process dependent on the nature of the antigen, its dose and form, and the location of the B-cell–antigen encounter.[19] B1 plasma cells express low affinity antibodies, usually of the IgM, IgA, or IgG3 subclass, that can bind to PRRs present on many pathogens. B2 cells are the primary producers of IgG1 and IgG2. Although most antigen-specific plasma cells will die after the infection has been resolved, a small portion will persist as memory cells that have the capacity to survive for many years. Secondary encounter with the same antigen results in the secretion of a high titer of antibodies with increased affinity.[18,19]

Because T cells can recognize microbial antigens only in association with host MHC molecules, free virus particles or bacteria are invisible to them. Thus, antibody provides the host's only specific defense against microbial organisms that are not cell associated. The importance of preexisting antibody in protective immunity against infectious diseases cannot be overemphasized. Antibody is likely to be the sole mechanism of protection against bacteria and parasites that have an exclusively extracellular lifestyle.

Memory

Immunologic memory is the ability of the immune system to respond with greater vigor to a reencounter with the same pathogen, and constitutes the basis for vaccination.[20] In the B-cell system, immediate protection is mediated by long-lived plasma cells that

Table 2
Characteristics of antibody isotypes

Antibody Isotype	Location	Function	Proportion of Total (%)
IgA	Mucosal areas such as the nasal passages, gut, respiratory tract, and urogenital tracts; also found in saliva, tears, and blood	Protects exposed surfaces of the body	10–15
IgD	Stomach and chest lining	Activates basophils and mast cells to produce antimicrobial agents	0.3
IgE	Lungs, skin, and mucous membranes	Initiate responses to allergens (ie, degranulation by mast cells); also implicated in defense against helminthes and protozoan parasites	0.02
IgG	All bodily fluids	Primary isotype responsible for clearing bacterial and viral infection; crosses placenta to confer passive immunity to neonates	75–85
IgM	Blood and lymph fluid	First antibody produced in response to a primary infection; activate immune mediators	5–10

secrete antibodies in an antigen-independent fashion and thus maintain constant antibody titers in serum and body fluids.[21] In response to antigenic stimulation, memory B cells rapidly proliferate and differentiate, resulting in a marked but brief increase in serum antibody levels.[22] The T-cell system is similarly divided between T-cell subsets that offer immediate and delayed protection.[23] Circulating or tissue-resident effector memory T (Tem) cells assess the body's frontline barriers and diseased tissues for foreign substances, and provide immediate effector function on antigen recognition.[23] By contrast, recall responses are mediated by central memory T (Tcm) cells that survey T-cell areas of the lymph nodes, and spleen and undergo rapid proliferation in response to antigen presented by DCs. Of importance, memory T and B cells as well as long-lived plasma cells are maintained at relatively constant numbers for the lifetime of the host, even in the absence of the specific antigen.[24–26] The section "Quantifying the immune response to vaccines" describes ways in which the immune response is measured to achieve the best protection from vaccines, as well as individual factors that affect the immune system's ability to function.

CREATING AN EFFECTIVE IMMUNE RESPONSE TO VACCINES

Many scientists and physicians have dedicated their lives to understanding the human immune response to infectious organisms against which effective vaccines have still not been developed. Although vaccines are studied intensively before licensure, insight into important aspects of vaccine performance and the success of immunization programs and policies can only be detected after vaccines enter widespread use. In addition, the understanding of epidemiologic principles such as herd immunity is critical.[27–29] For scientists to develop vaccines that are not simply an attenuated version of the wild-type pathogen, they must first understand the type of immune response required to effectively clear a particular infection. Because humoral responses are easier to measure and require less expensive equipment and research than T-cell responses, antibody levels are typically used as an indicator of the strength of an immune response.[5,28] However, for infectious agents that primarily elicit cellular immune responses, antibodies may not be the most accurate indicator of immunity.

Adjuvants

When vaccination with a live attenuated variant of the targeted pathogen is not an option, inactivated pathogens are used (see **Table 1**). Most inactivated vaccines have additional components known as adjuvants (from the Latin *adjuvare*, to help), which indirectly boost T-cell and B-cell responses by engaging components of the innate immune system.[30] Boosting immunity has many clinical advantages: (1) enhancing herd immunity by increasing vaccine responsiveness in the general population, (2) increasing seroconversion rates in individuals who have weakened immune responses as a result of advanced age or disease, (3) allowing the use of smaller doses of antigen (a point that is particularly important when large-scale vaccination is required such as in the case of H1N1), and (4) permitting immunization with fewer doses of vaccine and thereby reducing issues of compliance and logistics. In recent years, adjuvants have been shown to not only boost the immune response but also to direct the type of adaptive response required for a specific pathogen. Altering the immune response has its own clinical advantages: (1) providing functionally appropriate types of immune responses (Th1 vs Th2, CD8 vs CD4, specific antibody isotypes), (2) enhancing the generation of T-cell memory, (3) increasing the speed of the initial response, which may be critical during a pandemic outbreak, and (4) altering the breadth, specificity, and/or affinity of the response.[30,31]

Safety concerns for adjuvants

The adoption of new adjuvants into licensed vaccines has been slowed by a variety of hypothetical safety concerns, the most prominent of which is the increased risk of autoimmune disease. These concerns are based on observations that particular infections can trigger or exacerbate autoimmune disease by activating elements of the innate response. For example, Type 1 interferons are important in the pathogenesis of lupus, and disease flares are often triggered by subsequent viral infections.[32] PRR ligands have also been shown to break tolerance in animal models by suppressing regulatory T cells.[32] It should be noted, however, that adjuvants are engineered to enhance the response to immunogenic nonself antigens and few, if any, provide all of the stimuli needed to render a self-antigen sufficiently immunogenic to trigger autoimmunity.

QUANTIFYING THE IMMUNE RESPONSE TO VACCINES

Antibody Titers

The majority of immune responses to vaccines are measured by antibody testing.[1] However, there is a wide variety of antibody tests, including those that test a patient sample (usually serum) for the presence or absence of a specific antibody (qualitative) and those that measure that amount of antibody (quantitative). A summary of the most common antibody tests is shown in **Table 3**. Of importance is that many of these tests are not necessarily interchangeable between infection types, which was clearly demonstrated following an outbreak of varicella among health care workers at a large teaching hospital. A latex bead agglutination assay used to prescreen the workers was

Table 3
Common tests used to measure antibody responses

Diagnostic Method	Application	Strengths	Limitations
Agglutination	• Assesses the reaction of an antibody with an antigen by observing agglutination (clumping) of the antigen • Measures seroconversion following disease or vaccination • Assesses bacterial infections	Easy to perform	Semiquantitative
Radioimmunoassay (RIA)	• Radioactive label binds either antigen or antibody • Measures the radioactivity associated with the immune complex being tested	Quantitative	Requires a radioactivity license and trained staff
Enzyme-linked-immunosorbent serologic assay (ELISA)	• Measures an enzymatic reaction to an immune complex • Usually reported as geometric mean titers	Easy to perform Reliable Highly specific Established in clinical research	Requires expensive equipment Can only detect one antigen at a time Dependent on technician skills
Immunofluorescence (IFA)	• Labeling of antigens or antibodies with fluorescent dyes (can be either direct or indirect)	Fast Economical Can use several different antibodies or antigens on the same sample	Sensitive to photobleaching Subjective readout Dependent on technician skills

later associated with a high rate of false positivity, especially as compared with an IgG enzyme-linked immunosorbent assay.[33]

The ability of an antibody test to effectively detect the presence of antibody in a sample is dependent on the following qualities of the antibody.

1. Affinity: the binding strength between an antibody and antigen. Affinity directly affects the stability of an antibody-antigen complex and the ease with which this complex can be detected.
2. Avidity: the combined strength of bond affinities in an antibody-antigen complex. Reactions between multivalent antigens and antibodies have more avidity and are thus easier to detect. Strong avidity indicates a primary infection. Thus, tests for avidity have been important in determining which individuals may require extra doses of vaccines.[33,34]
3. Specificity: the attraction of an antibody to some antigenic determinants and not others. Detection insures that an antigen-specific response has been mounted.

Vaccines with the most immunogenic success have been obtained when the microbe has a bacteremic or viremic phase during which it is susceptible to the action of neutralizing antibodies. This phase must occur before the pathogen begins to replicate in the particular tissue or organ for which it has tropism. Examples include the vaccines against measles, mumps, rubella, varicella, hepatitis A (HAV), and hepatitis B (HBV).[2,4]

Reasons for Measuring the Immune Response

To establish the vaccine dose number required for immunity

Postlicensure studies of many vaccines have shown that while one dose is enough to prime the immune system, it is insufficient to prevent a modified "breakthrough" form of the disease. In multicenter clinical trials for varicella vaccine, for example, 12% of individuals failed to achieve protective antibody levels after 1 dose, and modified varicella disease was prevalent. After 2 doses, however, fewer than 1% of individuals failed to achieve a protective level antibody titer and the incidence of vaccine failures decreased significantly.[35,36] Similarly, measles outbreaks in the late 1980s demonstrated that one vaccine dose was not enough to prevent infection. Studies confirmed that a second dose achieved a higher degree of immunity and provided a "catch up" opportunity for unvaccinated individuals. It is unfortunate that more recent measles outbreaks have been caused by parents' failure to vaccinate their children as a result of fears about vaccine safety.[29]

To assess whether a cell-mediated immune response has been established

Cell-mediated immunity (CMI) is typically measured using T-Lymphocyte Proliferation or ELISpot assays. Because lysis of virally infected cells by cytotoxic T lymphocytes is an important component of the host immune response to many viral pathogens, CMI can be measured in response to several of the live virus vaccines, including measles, mumps, rubella, varicella, nasal influenza, oral polio, oral rotavirus, and yellow fever. Such measurements have helped in establishing dose number and in predicting the longevity of the immune response. The downside is that many CMI assays are performed in research laboratories and are not available in the commercial sector.

The varicella zoster virus (VZV)-specific lymphocyte cell proliferation assay has been used to establish correlations between the presence of virus-specific CMI and the occurrence of clinical disease. Healthy children who develop VZV-specific lymphocyte proliferation after the viral exanthem have mild primary VZV infection, whereas immunodeficient children who fail to have VZV-specific lymphocyte proliferation develop progressive disseminated varicella. Memory T lymphocytes can be boosted by exposure to disease or vaccination, which helps to explain why second episodes of herpes zoster (HZ) are rare in healthy individuals.[37] Similar observations have been made following vaccination against tetanus, diphtheria, pertussis, pneumococcus, meningococcus, and human papilloma virus.[1,4,28] CMI responses to HBV are often measured by ELISpot. This test provides a more reliable prediction of whether a vaccinated individual who is exposed in a high-risk setting has effectively mounted both arms of the immune response (ie, T-cell and B-cell responses).[38] This aspect is particularly important if health care workers have been exposed.

To understand how the immune system is influenced by factors such as age and stress
Immune senescence (or the age-related decline in immune function), comorbid illness and, often, compromised nutrition put older individuals at increased risk of contracting infectious diseases such as influenza, pneumonia, urinary tract infections, and tuberculosis as well as their associated complications.[39,40] The reduction in immune responses is thought to be primarily related to the involution of the thymus and coincident drop in T-cell numbers and Th-cell–dependent antibody responses.[41] Antibody titer decreases of 50% and 75% are shown to occur by ages 50 and 75 years, respectively. For these reasons, it is more of a challenge to elicit effective immune responses to vaccination among older individuals. Thus, alternative adjuvants and/or additional vaccine doses are often recommended for this population.[42,43]

An immature immune system is similarly susceptible to infectious disease. Indeed, infants born very prematurely (ie, 28–32 weeks of gestation) have decreased maternal antibody titers because placental transfer does not begin until after week 28 of gestation.[44] Preterm newborns also have lower numbers of both CD4+ and CD8+ T cells and lack expression of important cell-surface receptors.[45] Despite having an immature immune system at birth, however, studies suggest that by the time preterm infants are 6 to 8 weeks old they are capable of developing an effective immune response to most vaccines, including tetanus, diphtheria, pertussis, polio, *Haemophilus influenzae* type B, meningococcus type C, and rotavirus. Thus, it is recommended that these vaccinations be given at the usual 2-month well visit and not on a delayed schedule.[46,47] This is a critical point to convey because studies over the last 15 years have shown that preterm infants in the United States and many European countries are still being immunized 1 to 2 months late, a finding that has been linked to deaths from pertussis and other infectious diseases.[47] To date, the only vaccine shown to be poorly immunogenic among preterm infants is HBV, explaining why current recommendations state that premature babies born to HBV-positive mothers should receive a fourth dose of the vaccine.[48]

The negative effect of physical and physiologic stress, as a result of everything from grief to academic examinations, to pain and disease, on immune function has been well documented by psychoneuroimmunologists.[49,50] Stress affects innate and adaptive immune responses, decreasing lymphocyte numbers, natural killer cell function, and cytokine production, and increasing an individual's risk of both developing infectious disease and having a delayed recovery. Research has also shown that responses to both viral and bacterial vaccines are delayed and shorter lived in stressed individuals.[50]

SUMMARY

Many people, including primary care practitioners, public health officials, insurance and funding agents, academic and pharmaceutical researchers, parents, and teachers, are critical to the successful prevention of infectious disease. Given that many young parents and physicians have never witnessed the ravages of vaccine-preventable diseases, the authors hope this overview of the immune response to vaccines, including ways in which it is measured and/or augmented to enhance its effectiveness, will aid these individuals in their quest to reduce vaccine-preventable disease burdens around the world.

REFERENCES

1. Plotkin SA, Orenstein WA, Offit PA. Vaccines: expert consult. 5th edition. Philadephia (PA): Elsevier Health Sciences; 2008.
2. Plotkin SA. New vaccination strategies. Bull Acad Natl Med 2008;192(3):511–8 [discussion: 518–9] [in French].
3. Schuchat A, Bell BP. Monitoring the impact of vaccines postlicensure: new challenges, new opportunities. Expert Rev Vaccines 2008;7(4):437–56.
4. D'Argenio DA, Wilson CB. A decade of vaccines: Integrating immunology and vaccinology for rational vaccine design. Immunity 2010;33(4):437–40.
5. Centers for Disease Control and Prevention. Epidemiology and prevention of vaccine-preventable diseases. In: Wolfe S, Atkinson W, Hamborsky J, et al, editors. Epidemiology & Prevention of Vaccine Preventable Diseases. 11th edition. Washington, DC: Public Health Foundation; 2009.
6. Beutler B. Microbe sensing, positive feedback loops, and the pathogenesis of inflammatory diseases. Immunol Rev 2009;227(1):248–63.
7. Takeuchi O, Akira S. Pattern recognition receptors and inflammation. Cell 2010; 140(6):805–20.
8. Banchereau J, Briere F, Caux C, et al. Immunobiology of dendritic cells. Annu Rev Immunol 2000;18:767–811.
9. Jenkins MK, Khoruts A, Ingulli E, et al. In vivo activation of antigen-specific CD4 T cells. Annu Rev Immunol 2001;19:23–45.
10. Campbell JJ, Butcher EC. Chemokines in tissue-specific and microenvironment-specific lymphocyte homing. Curr Opin Immunol 2000;12(3):336–41.
11. Wong P, Pamer EG. Feedback regulation of pathogen-specific T cell priming. Immunity 2003;18(4):499–511.
12. Harty JT, Tvinnereim AR, White DW. CD8+ T cell effector mechanisms in resistance to infection. Annu Rev Immunol 2000;18:275–308.
13. Watts C. Capture and processing of exogenous antigens for presentation on MHC molecules. Annu Rev Immunol 1997;15:821–50.
14. Reiner SL. Decision making during the conception and career of CD4+ T cells. Nat Rev Immunol 2009;9(2):81–2.
15. Lenardo M, Chan KM, Hornung F, et al. Mature T lymphocyte apoptosis—immune regulation in a dynamic and unpredictable antigenic environment. Annu Rev Immunol 1999;17:221–53.
16. Dutton RW, Bradley LM, Swain SL. T cell memory. Annu Rev Immunol 1998;16: 201–23.
17. Sandel PC, Monroe JG. Negative selection of immature B cells by receptor editing or deletion is determined by site of antigen encounter. Immunity 1999;10(3): 289–99.
18. Manz RA, Hauser AE, Hiepe F, et al. Maintenance of serum antibody levels. Annu Rev Immunol 2005;23:367–86.
19. Shapiro-Shelef M, Calame K. Regulation of plasma-cell development. Nat Rev Immunol 2005;5(3):230–42.

20. Ahmed R, Gray D. Immunological memory and protective immunity: understanding their relation. Science 1996;272(5258):54–60.
21. Moser K, Tokoyoda K, Radbruch A, et al. Stromal niches, plasma cell differentiation and survival. Curr Opin Immunol 2006;18(3):265–70.
22. Pelletier N, McHeyzer-Williams MG. B cell memory: how to start and when to end. Nat Immunol 2009;10(12):1233–5.
23. Sallusto F, Geginat J, Lanzavecchia A. Central memory and effector memory T cell subsets: function, generation, and maintenance. Annu Rev Immunol 2004; 22:745–63.
24. Doherty PC, Hou S, Tripp RA. CD8+ T-cell memory to viruses. Curr Opin Immunol 1994;6(4):545–52.
25. Lau LL, Jamieson BD, Somasundraram T, et al. Cytotoxic T-cell memory without antigen. Nature 1994;369(6482):648–52.
26. Deliyannis G, Jackson DC, Ede NJ, et al. Induction of long-term memory CD8(+) T cells for recall of viral clearing responses against influenza virus. J Virol 2002; 76(9):4212–21.
27. Alam R. A brief review of the immune system. Prim Care 1998;25(4):727–38.
28. de Quadros CA, Andrus JK, editors. Recent advances in immunization. 2nd edition. Pan American Health Organization; 2006.
29. Offit PA, Moser CA. The problem with Dr Bob's alternative vaccine schedule. Pediatrics 2009;123(1):e164–9.
30. Kenney RT, Cross AS. Adjuvants for the future. In: Levine MM, Good MF, Liu MA, et al, editors. New generation vaccines. New York: Informa Healthcare USA, Inc; 2010. p. 250–62.
31. Coffman RL, Sher A, Seder RA. Vaccine adjuvants: putting innate immunity to work. Immunity 2010;33(4):492–503.
32. Zandman-Goddard G, Shoenfeld Y. Infections and SLE. Autoimmunity 2005; 38(7):473–85.
33. Behrman A, Schmid DS, Crivaro A, et al. A cluster of primary varicella cases among healthcare workers with false-positive varicella zoster virus titers. Infect Control Hosp Epidemiol 2003;24(3):202–6.
34. Prince HE, Leber AL. Validation of an in-house assay for cytomegalovirus immunoglobulin G (CMV IgG) avidity and relationship of avidity to CMV IgM levels. Clin Diagn Lab Immunol 2002;9(4):824–7.
35. Watson B. Humoral and cell-mediated immune responses in children and adults after 1 and 2 doses of varicella vaccine. J Infect Dis 2008; 197(Suppl 2):S143–6.
36. Arvin AM. Humoral and cellular immunity to varicella-zoster virus: an overview. J Infect Dis 2008;197(Suppl 2):S58–60.
37. Arvin AM. Varicella-zoster virus. Clin Microbiol Rev 1996;9(3):361–81.
38. Cassidy WM, Watson B, Ioli VA, et al. A randomized trial of alternative two- and three-dose hepatitis B vaccination regimens in adolescents: antibody responses, safety, and immunologic memory. Pediatrics 2001;107(4):626–31.
39. Kay MM, Makinodan T. Relationship between aging and immune system. Prog Allergy 1981;29:134–81.
40. Schneider EL. Infectious diseases in the elderly. Ann Intern Med 1983;98(3): 395–400.
41. Aspinall R, Pitts D, Lapenna A, et al. Immunity in the elderly: the role of the thymus. J Comp Pathol 2010;142(Suppl 1):S111–5.
42. Centers for Disease Control and Prevention (CDC). Licensure of a high-dose inactivated influenza vaccine for persons aged > or = 65 years (Fluzone High-Dose)

and guidance for use—United States, 2010. MMWR Morb Mortal Wkly Rep 2010; 59(16):485–6.
43. Guy B. Strategies to improve the effect of vaccination in the elderly: the vaccine producer's perspective. J Comp Pathol 2010;142(Suppl 1):S133–7.
44. Roberton DM, Marshall H, Dinan L, et al. Developmental immunology and vaccines: immune responses to vaccines in premature infants. Expert Rev Vaccines 2004;3(4):343–7.
45. D'Angio CT. Active immunization of premature and low birth-weight infants: a review of immunogenicity, efficacy, and tolerability. Paediatr Drugs 2007;9(1): 17–32.
46. The Committee on the Infectious Diseases of the American Academy of Pediatrics. Recommended childhood immunization schedule. In: Peter G, editor. Red book: report of the Committee on Infectious Diseases. Elk Grove Village (IL): American Academy of Pediatrics; 1994.
47. Siegrist CA. Vaccination strategies for children with specific medical conditions: a paediatrician's viewpoint. Eur J Pediatr 1997;156(12):899–904.
48. Ballesteros-Trujillo A, et al. Response to hepatitis B vaccine in preterm infants: four-dose schedule. Am J Perinatol 2001;18(7):379–85.
49. Kiecolt-Glaser JK, et al. Psychoneuroimmunology: psychological influences on immune function and health. J Consult Clin Psychol 2002;70(3):537–47.
50. Glaser R, Kiecolt-Glaser JK. Stress-induced immune dysfunction: implications for health. Nat Rev Immunol 2005;5(3):243–51.

Routine Pediatric Immunization, Special Cases in Pediatrics: Prematurity, Chronic Disease, Congenital Heart Disease: Recent Advancements/Changes in Pediatric Vaccines

Daniel Walmsley, DO

KEYWORDS

• Childhood pediatric immunizations • Prematurity
• Respiratory syncytial virus • Palivizumab (Synagis)

GENERAL PRINCIPLES

The routine immunization of children is a startling success story for preventive primary care. Through the standard vaccination of children, there has been a dramatic decrease in several serious infections. For example, the adoption of the *Haemophilus influenzae* type B (HiB) vaccine has reduced diseases caused by *H influenzae* by 98%.[1] Recently the introduction of pneumococcal conjugate vaccine and now expansion from 7 to 13 valents has lead to a significant decrease in invasive pneumococcal disease.[2] Overall, the routine immunization of children has led to a dramatic improvement in the health of children.

Vaccine Schedules

The field of immunizations is constantly evolving, with new and improved vaccines arriving on a regular basis. Immunization guidelines are continuously updated and revised by the Centers for Disease Control and Prevention (CDC), the Advisory Committee on Immunization Practices (ACIP), the Committee of Infectious Diseases

The authors have nothing to disclose.
Division of General Pediatrics, Thomas Jefferson University/Nemours Pediatrics, 833 Chestnut Street Suite 300, Philadelphia, PA 19107, USA
E-mail address: dwalmsle@nemours.org

Prim Care Clin Office Pract 38 (2011) 595–609
doi:10.1016/j.pop.2011.07.002 **primarycare.theclinics.com**

of the American Academy of Pediatrics (AAP), and the American Academy of Family Physicians (AAFP) (**Fig. 1**). A recommended immunization schedule for children and adolescents who start late or are behind on vaccinations, the "catch-up schedule," is also updated on a regular basis (**Fig. 2**). The catch-up schedule also describes minimum intervals between doses that can be used for special circumstances to accelerate vaccination, such as for children who are behind or who have impending travel plans.

The annual immunization recommendations and catch-up schedules are updated every January and are widely available online and in print. The vaccine recommendations are based on risk of exposure and burden of disease in combination with any possible adverse event of a particular vaccine or vaccine constituent.

Vaccine Coverage Rates

Immunization rates have steadily increased over the last few decades. Current vaccine coverage rates for universally accepted routine vaccines range from 40% to between 38% and 94% (**Table 1**).[3] This increase can be attributed to multiple public health and legislative endeavors such as the comprehensive enforcement of school and state laws, provider education, and availability of centralized immunization records. Healthy People 2010 set a coverage-level goal of 90% for all children, so work is still necessary to ensure high coverage rates.[4] For primary care providers, there are a few additional methods that can be undertaken to further increase the coverage level. As physicians we can advocate for the adoption of a centralized registry of immunizations for all patients. Multiple studies have shown that centralized immunization records have led to an increase in vaccine coverage rates among children.[5] Clinicians also can work to remove barriers associated with vaccination by checking the immunization

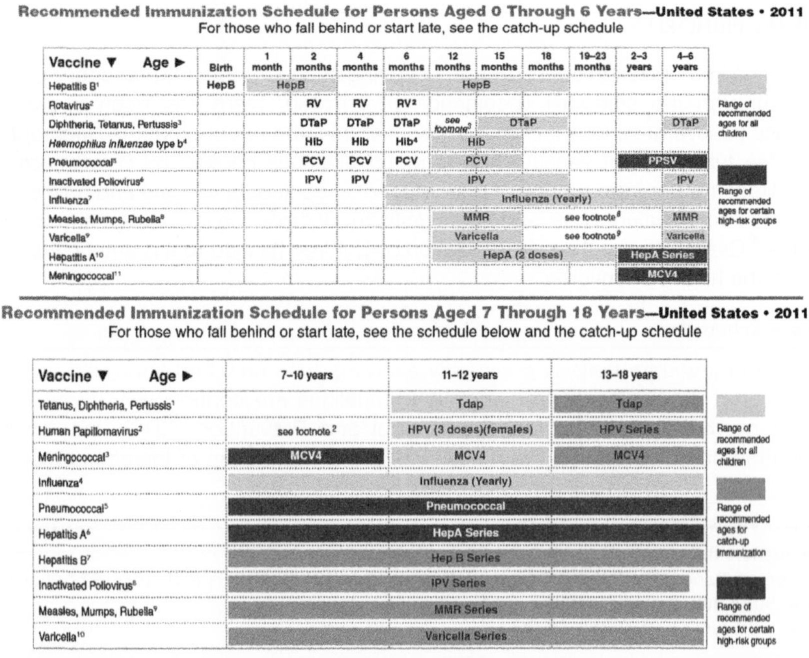

Fig. 1. Recommended immunization schedule for persons aged 0 through 18 years: United States, 2011. The catch-up schedule is shown in **Fig. 2**.

Catch-up Immunization Schedule for Persons Aged 4 Months Through 18 Years Who Start Late or Who Are More Than 1 Month Behind—United States • 2011

The table below provides catch-up schedules and minimum intervals between doses for children whose vaccinations have been delayed. A vaccine series does not need to be restarted, regardless of the time that has elapsed between doses. Use the section appropriate for the child's age

Vaccine	Minimum Age for Dose 1	Minimum Interval Between Doses: Dose 1 to Dose 2	Dose 2 to Dose 3	Dose 3 to Dose 4	Dose 4 to Dose 5
PERSONS AGED 4 MONTHS THROUGH 6 YEARS					
Hepatitis B[1]	Birth	4 weeks	8 weeks (and at least 16 weeks after first dose)		
Rotavirus[2]	6 wks	4 weeks	4 weeks[2]		
Diphtheria, Tetanus, Pertussis[3]	6 wks	4 weeks	4 weeks	6 months	6 months[3]
Haemophilus influenzae type b[4]	6 wks	4 weeks if first dose administered at younger than age 12 months 8 weeks (as final dose) if first dose administered at age 12–14 months No further doses needed if first dose administered at age 15 months or older	4 weeks[4] if current age is younger than 12 months 8 weeks (as final dose)[4] if current age is 12 months or older and first dose administered at younger than age 12 months and second dose administered at younger than 15 months No further doses needed if previous dose administered at age 15 months or older	8 weeks (as final dose) This dose only necessary for children aged 12 months through 59 months who received 3 doses before age 12 months	
Pneumococcal[5]	6 wks	4 weeks if first dose administered at younger than age 12 months 8 weeks (as final dose for healthy children) if first dose administered at age 12 months or older or current age 24 through 59 months No further doses needed for healthy children if first dose administered at age 24 months or older	4 weeks if current age is younger than 12 months 8 weeks (as final dose for healthy children) if current age is 12 months or older No further doses needed for healthy children if previous dose administered at age 24 months or older	8 weeks (as final dose) This dose only necessary for children aged 12 months through 59 months who received 3 doses before age 12 months or for children at high risk who received 3 doses at any age	
Inactivated Poliovirus[6]	6 wks	4 weeks	4 weeks	6 months[6]	
Measles, Mumps, Rubella[7]	12 mos	4 weeks			
Varicella[8]	12 mos	3 months			
Hepatitis A[9]	12 mos	6 months			
PERSONS AGED 7 THROUGH 18 YEARS					
Tetanus, Diphtheria/ Tetanus, Diphtheria, Pertussis[10]	7 yrs[10]	4 weeks	4 weeks if first dose administered at younger than age 12 months 6 months if first dose administered at 12 months or older	6 months if first dose administered at younger than age 12 months	
Human Papillomavirus[11]	9 yrs	Routine dosing intervals are recommended (females)[11]			
Hepatitis A[9]	12 mos	6 months			
Hepatitis B[1]	Birth	4 weeks	8 weeks (and at least 16 weeks after first dose)		
Inactivated Poliovirus[6]	6 wks	4 weeks	4 weeks[6]	6 months[6]	
Measles, Mumps, Rubella[7]	12 mos	4 weeks			
Varicella[8]	12 mos	3 months if person is younger than age 13 years 4 weeks if person is aged 13 years or older			

Fig. 2. Catch-up immunization schedule for persons aged 4 months through 18 years who start late or who are more than 1 month behind schedule: United States, 2011.

Table 1
Reported vaccine coverage rates for the United States (2008–2009) and healthy people 2020 goals

Vaccine	Number of Doses by Age 19–35 months	Vaccine Coverage Rates, 2008 (%)	Healthy People 2020 Coverage Level Goal (%)
DTaP	4	85	90
HiB	3	57[a]	90
Hepatitis B	3	94	90
IPV	3	94	90
PCV	4	80	90
MMR	1	92	90
Varicella	1	91	90
Hepatitis A	2	40	60
Rotavirus	2 (or more)[b]	38[a]	80

Abbreviations: DTaP, diphtheria, tetanus, and pertussis; HiB, *Haemophilus influenzae* type B; IPV, inactivated poliovirus vaccine; MMR, measles, mumps, and rubella; PCV, pneumococcal conjugate vaccine.

[a] Data from first and second quarters of 2009.

[b] Number depends on type of vaccine (Rotarix (2 doses) versus Rotateq (3 doses) used).

status of patients at every visit and vaccinating even during acute-care visits. All vaccines can be given even in the presence of mild illness. This concept of vaccination at acute-care visits can at times be controversial. One study showed that vaccination at acute visits actually decreased the number of patients who attended 18-month well-child visits.[6] Despite this fact, clinicians should consider any opportunity to vaccinate children against disease and, in general, vaccinating at acute visits can help achieve the goal of improved vaccination coverage levels.

Vaccine Interchangeability

The ACIP and AAP recommend that, when feasible, the same vaccine should be used for the primary series but that multiple doses of any vaccine are sufficient, including rotavirus.[7] The interchangeability of most vaccines produced by different manufacturers to prevent the same disease is supported by multiple studies. One such study showed that the 3-dose series using different HiB conjugate vaccines equaled or exceeded the response when the same vaccine was used for the series.[7] Despite this recommendation, data in this area are limited, especially the case of diphtheria, tetanus, and pertussis vaccine (DTaP). As a result, it is best to use the same vaccine for the primary series whenever possible.

Vaccine Safety

The National Childhood Vaccine Injury Act was passed in 1986. This act created a compensation program for families with children affected by vaccine-associated adverse events.[8] The CDC and Food and Drug Administration (FDA) jointly operate a system called Vaccine Adverse Event Reporting System (VAERS) to detect early warning signals and generate hypothesis about possible new vaccine adverse events. This system can be accessed online at http://www.cdc.gov/vaccines/pubs/acip-list.htmor by calling 800-822-7967. A success story of this system came in 1999, when reports of intussusception related to a new rotavirus vaccine was identified after adverse events were detected in the VAERS. This vaccine is no longer available in the United States. In addition, informed consent and the education of parents regarding vaccines have been identified as a critical part of vaccine safety, and are required by The National Childhood Vaccine Act of 1986. In response, Vaccine Information Statements (VIS) have been created by the CDC and National Vaccine Advisory Committee. These statements describe the diseases that vaccines are intended to prevent, the risks and benefits of the vaccines, and the procedure for reporting adverse events and/or seeking compensation for a vaccine adverse event.[7] The VIS should be given to parents at every administration of vaccines to children, and are available on the CDC's Web site or through a public health office.

ROUTINE CHILDHOOD VACCINES

Hepatitis B

The acquisition of hepatitis B infection at a younger age is associated with a stronger probability of developing chronic hepatitis B infection, cirrhosis, or cancer. Therefore, all children between the ages of 0 and 18 years should be vaccinated against hepatitis B. The first dose must be a monovalent vaccine given to all newborn infants before discharge from the hospital. After the birth dose, the series can be completed using 2 doses of single-antigen vaccines or up to 3 doses of combination vaccines. The minimum interval between doses is 4 weeks between the first 2 doses and 2 months, but preferably 4 to 6 months between the second and third doses. Typically the vaccine is given at birth, followed by dose 2 between 1 and 2 months of age and dose 3 between 6 and 18 months of age (most commonly at age 6 months) (see **Fig. 1**). Hepatitis B vaccines come in monovalent single antigens called Recombivax HB and Engerix-B. The two currently available pediatric hepatitis B combination vaccines include Comvax (Hepatitis and HiB) and Pediarix (Hepatitis B, DTaP, and inactivated poliovirus vaccine [IPV]). Comvax and Pediarix are approved for ages 2, 4, and 12 to 15 months. Response to the vaccine in all age groups is excellent in all age groups, with antihepatitis antibodies present in 85% to 99% of recipients.[9] A special circumstance for hepatitis B vaccination exists for premature infants.

Maternal Hepatitis B Status

Routine screening of all pregnant women for hepatitis B surface antigen (HBsAg) is mandatory because infants born to HBsAg-positive mothers require the administration of the hepatitis B vaccine and hepatitis B immune globulin (HBIG) in a timely manner. Infants born to mothers who are HBSAg-positive need to receive their hepatitis B vaccine and HBIG within 12 hours of life. Infants born to mothers who are hepatitis B status unknown need to receive their hepatitis B vaccine within 12 hours but have a period of 7 days after birth before HBIG is required. As a result, the HBsAg status of the mother can be determined within the first week of life. If she is negative, HIBIG may be withheld.[10] HBIG is a blood product and is a reason to delay administration if maternal HBsAg status can be determined. However, due to follow-up concerns and issues of availability of HBIG outside the hospital setting, immune globulin should be given before hospital discharge for these infants if the mother's status cannot be determined during that hospital stay. Any infant born to a mother who is HBsAg-positive should also receive an additional dose of hepatitis B vaccine at 1 month of age.[7]

HiB

The advent of universal HiB vaccination for all children has led to a dramatic reduction in the incidence of invasive HiB diseases among children. By 2000, the number of cases in children of invasive HiB disease declined by greater than 99%. HiB vaccination is recommended for all infants starting at 6 weeks to 2 months of age (see **Fig. 1**).

There are several conjugate vaccines available that differ in their carrier proteins and number of dosages required for the primary series. Primary series of HiB for infants can consist of a 2-dose or 3-dose vaccine schedule. The HiB conjugate vaccines, called HiB PRP-T or HbOC, can be used for a 3-dose vaccine schedule given at recommended 2-month intervals between the ages of 6 weeks and 6 months. A minimum of 1 month can be observed for these vaccines. The PRP-OMP conjugate vaccine is given as a 2-dose series separated by 2-month intervals. A booster vaccine is required between the ages of 12 to 15 months of age for both the 3-dose and 2-dose series.[7] A combination DTaP-HiB vaccine (TriHIBit) is available and is approved as a booster dose only. Multiple studies have shown that giving different HiB vaccines during the primary series induces a response similar to that induced by the primary series with the same vaccine, and that booster doses with different vaccines induce even stronger responses.

Pneumococcal Conjugate and Polysaccharide Vaccines

Since the introduction of pneumococcal conjugate vaccine, there has been a dramatic reduction in the incidence of invasive and noninvasive pneumococcal disease. In 2010, a 13-valent pneumococcal conjugate vaccine, Prevnar 13 (PCV13) was licensed by the FDA and subsequently, its usage was recommended by the ACIP and AAP. This vaccine contains the same serotypes as PCV7 plus 6 additional serotypes, and was found to induce a comparative response in those children immunized with PCV7. The AAP and ACIP recommend the routine vaccination of all children aged 2 to 59 months with PCV13, vaccination of children aged 60 to 71 months with underlying medical conditions that increase their risk for pneumococcal disease (**Table 2**), and PCV13 vaccination for children who previously received one or more doses of PCV7.[11]

Based on the new recommendations, PCV13 is to replace PCV7 and is to be given at the same schedule; 4 doses: 2, 4, 6, and 12 to 15 months (see **Fig. 1**). Fewer dosages are required if the child begins the schedule at 7 months of age or older

Table 2
Underlying medical conditions that are indications for pneumococcal vaccination among children, by risk group

Risk Group	Condition
Immunocompetent children	Chronic heart disease Chronic lung disease Diabetes mellitus Cerebrospinal fluid leaks Cochlear implant
Children with functional or anatomic asplenia	Sickle cell disease and other hemoglobinopathies Congenital or acquired asplenia, or splenic dysfunction
Children with immunocompromising conditions	HIV infection Chronic renal failure and nephrotic syndrome Diseases associated with treatment with immunosuppressive drugs or radiation therapy, including malignant neoplasms, leukemias, lymphomas and Hodgkin disease; or solid organ transplantation Congenital immunodeficiency

Abbreviation: HIV, human immunodeficiency virus.
Data from Advisory Committee on Immunization Practices, 2011.

(see **Fig. 2**). Children who received one or more doses of PCV7 should complete their immunization series with PCV13, with at least one dose of PCV13 given to children between the ages of 12 and 23 months. A single supplemental dose of PCV13 is recommended for all children aged 24 to 59 months who have received 4 doses of PCV7. Children with certain underlying medical conditions (see **Table 2**) who have received 3 doses of PCV (7 or 13) should receive a single dose of PCV13 before 71 months. PCV13 is not recommended routinely for healthy children who are 5 years or older.[12]

DTaP

Diphtheria, tetanus, and pertussis are 3 diseases that can cause significant morbidity and mortality in children. While cases of all 3 have decreased significantly over the years thanks to vaccines, there are still sporadic infections and they remain a risk to children. Immunization of children and adolescents to prevent these diseases is completed with a vaccine composed of diphtheria and tetanus toxoids combined with an acellular pertussis component. Before 1992 whole-cell DTP was the only pertussis vaccine available but, due to the relatively high rate of adverse reactions, the vaccine was changed to a newer acellular pertussis.[7]

Immunization with DTaP vaccine is recommended for all children younger than 7 years. Primary vaccination consists of 3 doses of DTaP vaccine given at 2, 4, and 6 months of age (see **Fig. 1**). The minimum age to start the vaccine series is 6 weeks and the minimum interval between doses is 4 weeks. Two booster dosages are recommended at between 15 and 18 months of age, and at school entry between 4 and 6 years of age.[13]

IPV

Infection with poliovirus, which was at one time a common disease, is now nonexistent in the United States, with the last indigenously transmitted case occurring in 1979. There are still cases of poliomyelitis in multiple countries worldwide, although we are closer to global eradication of poliomyelitis.[14] Vaccination against poliomyelitis is recommended for all children. Previously, vaccination occurred with a live attenuated oral polio vaccine (OPV). In 2000, recommendations were switched to the exclusive use of enhanced IPV in the United States because of the association of vaccine-associated paralytic poliomyelitis in people who received OPV. OPV is still available worldwide and is the most commonly used polio vaccine in the world. OPV continues to be the preferred vaccine in countries where poliomyelitis is or recently was endemic, and it is the only vaccine suitable for eradication of the disease.[7]

IPV is recommended to be given at 2, 4, and 6 to 18 months of age. It can be given as early as 6 weeks and has a minimum interval of 4 weeks. A booster dose of IPV is recommended before school entry between 4 and 6 years of age. (see **Fig. 1**) With some combination vaccines, children may get an additional dose of IPV at 12 to 15 months of age; this booster does not count toward their primary series and has not been shown to cause any adverse effects.[15]

Rotavirus

Rotavirus is the single most important viral cause of severe gastroenteritis in children worldwide. In developing countries it is a major cause of childhood death. Nearly every child in the United States is infected with rotavirus by the age of 5 years, with most developing gastroenteritis. Although death from rotavirus in the United States is rare (20–70 cases per year), many cases of rotavirus result in significant dehydration and the need for hospitalization. As a result, the development of a rotavirus vaccine has been important in decreasing the burden of this disease.

In 1999, an oral rotavirus vaccine called Rotashield was recommended for universal vaccination of infants but was removed from the market within 1 year, due to an epidemiologic link to intussusception.[16] Two oral rotavirus vaccines were subsequently developed and released in 2006. These vaccines had extensive preclinical trials to determine whether there was any link to intussusception. In both studies, no increase in intussusception was noted among receipts of the vaccines versus placebo.[17]

The two currently licensed oral rotavirus vaccines are a monovalent vaccine (Rotarix) and a pentavalent reassortant vaccine (Rotateq). Both vaccines have shown similar efficacy in decreasing the development of severe gastroenteritis, emergency department visits, and hospitalizations caused by rotavirus. Rotarix is given as a 2-dose series at 2 and 4 months whereas Rotateq is given as a 3-dose series at 2, 4, and 6 months. Both vaccine series must be started before 15 weeks of age and the last dose must be given before 32 weeks of age. Previously there had been concern regarding viral shedding and the risk of infecting household members who may be immunocompromised. Subsequent studies have shown that there is a low risk for this infection, and infants in households with people who may have impaired immune systems for any reason may still receive the rotavirus vaccine.[7]

MMR

Vaccination has significantly reduced the incidence of measles, mumps, and rubella (MMR) infections in the United States. Measles causes approximately 20 to 30 cases per year, mumps causes sporadic small outbreaks, and rubella has been deemed no longer endemic in the United States.[18] The MMR vaccine consists of live attenuated viruses, and is given starting at 12 months of age (see **Fig. 1**). The vaccine produces 95% to 98% antibody coverage in recipients; however, occasional outbreaks of measles in schools due to importation, unimmunized children, or vaccine failure has necessitated the use of a booster MMR vaccine between 4 and 6 years of age. During outbreaks affecting children younger than 1 year or for any child travelling internationally before the age of 1 year, MMR can be given at 6 months of age. This dose of the vaccine should not be considered part of the primary series, and therefore the child should still receive MMR at 1 year of age.[7]

The MMR vaccine has been a subject of controversy regarding autism. Since the 1980s, the rate of autism has been increasing throughout the world, and many parents of autistic children and some professionals have identified a temporal association between immunizations and the onset of more evident symptoms of autism in the second year of life, specifically MMR. There has never been any evidence to support a link between MMR and autism.[19]

Varicella

Varicella vaccination has been available since March 1995. It has led to a significant decline in wild-type varicella infection. Varicella is a live attenuated vaccine given to children between 12 and 15 months of age. It has been found to be 95% effective in preventing severe varicella disease and 70% to 90% effective against mild to moderate disease.[7] Due to reported outbreaks of varicella and possible vaccine failures after a first dose, a booster varicella dose was recommended by the ACIP in 2006. This booster is recommended to be given between 4 and 6 years of age (see **Fig. 1**). In addition, the ACIP has also recommended that people older than 13 years without documented varicella infection should also receive the varicella vaccine as 2 doses separated by 4 to 8 weeks.[7] An MMRV combination vaccine is on the market but is not recommended for the 12- to 15-month dose, because of a reported twofold increase in febrile seizures. It is recommended for the 4- to 6-year booster, if available.

Hepatitis A

Hepatitis A vaccination had been recommended in states where the incidence of hepatitis A infection has been consistently elevated. In 2005, this recommendation was expanded throughout the nation when a dramatic decrease in hepatitis A was found in the states following the prior recommendation. All children should receive hepatitis A vaccine at 1 year of age followed by a booster given at a minimum of 6 months later. Unimmunized children older than the age of 2 years may receive the series. However, at present, catch-up is not universally recommended after the age of 2 unless the child lives in an endemic area.[20] Some states have programs encouraging the routine vaccination of children older than 2 years.

ADOLESCENT VACCINES

Meningococcal Conjugate Vaccine (Menactra)

A quadrivalent meningococcal diphtheria vaccine (MCV4) covering serogroups A, C, Y, and W-135 was introduced in January 2005. Along with TdaP, it ushered in a new era of adolescent vaccination. The vaccine covers the serogroups that cause approximately two-thirds of meningococcal disease that occurs in children 18 to 24 years of age. Infants and young children are more likely to be infected by the B serogroups; however, as of yet a successful vaccine to cover the B serogroup has not been developed, due to issues regarding the poor immunogenicity of the B capsular proteins in humans.[21]

The MCV4 vaccine is recommended for people between the ages of 11 and 21 years, adolescents at high school entry, and college freshmen (see **Fig. 1**). Recently a booster dose has been recommended by the ACIP because studies show that immunity toward MCV4 may wane by the ages of 16 to 21 years.[22] For persons receiving the vaccine between 11 and 15 years, one booster dose should be given between 16 and 18 years. As of now it is recommended that persons older than 16 who have not had the MCV4 vaccine should be given one dose. In the United States, vaccination for children younger than 11 years is currently under study, and most consider that the ACIP will soon recommend its usage in younger children.

TdaP

It has been shown that immunity toward diphtheria, tetanus, and pertussis continues to wane in adults. Specifically, young adults and adolescents were found to be the reservoirs for pertussis disease that was being transmitted to infants. As a result, a booster dose of TdaP is universally recommended starting at the age of 11 to 12 years.[23] The addition of acellular pertussis to the tetanus booster has been estimated to prevent between 1.3 million and 6.5 million cases of pertussis over a decade.[24]

Human Papillomavirus

Virtually all cases of cervical cancer and most cases of anal cancer are caused by viral infection with specific strains of human papillomavirus (HPV). Two vaccines against HPV, namely a quadrivalent (Gardasil) and bivalent vaccine (Cervarix), have been developed to vaccinate against HPV infection. In addition to protecting against cervical and anal cancer, the vaccines also protect against genital warts. Gardasil targets HPV types 16, 18, 6, and 11, whereas Cervarix targets HPV types 16 and 18. HPV types 16 and 18 cause about 70% of cervical cancer and about 50% of precancerous lesions. HPV types 6 and 11 cause 90% of genital warts.[25]

The ACIP recommend that HPV vaccination should be routinely offered to all females between the ages of 11 and 12 years. The vaccine can be given as early as

9 years of age. In 2009, the FDA approved the use of HPV vaccine in males and subsequently, the ACIP stated that it may be given to males between the ages of 9 and 26 years to reduce their likelihood of acquiring genital warts.[26] The rationale for giving HPV vaccine to males includes preventing the burden of genital warts and protecting females form infection. For homosexual males, it is especially important to vaccinate against HPV for the prevention of anal cancer. There is some controversy among providers about whether all males should receive the HPV vaccine; to date it has been listed as an optional vaccine by most professional organizations. Although most providers have responded by offering it as an "optional" vaccine to males, the author's experience has been that most males opt for the vaccine if given the choice.

The HPV vaccine is administered slightly differently based on the product given to the patient. Gardasil is administered in 3 doses, with 2 months in between doses 1 and 2 and then 6 months separating doses 1 and 3, whereas Cervarix is given in 3 doses with 1 month in between doses 1 and 2 and then 6 months separating doses 1 and 3. The vaccine series can start any time between the ages of 9 and 26 years. The vaccine's effectiveness is improved if administered before the onset of sexual activity, as the vaccine does not accelerate the clearance of a preexistent HPV infection.

CONTRAINDICATIONS

There are certain circumstances when a vaccine may be contraindicated, and at other times the vaccine may have a precaution meaning that the benefits and risks of the vaccine should be weighed before administration. Minor illnesses do not contraindicate vaccines, as there is no evidence for increased risk of adverse events or decreased immunogenicity with minor illness.[25] The only contraindication that is absolute among all vaccines is a history of anaphylaxis to a vaccine or any of its constituent parts. A summary of vaccine contraindications and adverse reactions appears in **Table 3**.

SPECIAL CASES IN PEDIATRICS: PREMATURITY

Hepatitis B Vaccine in Premature Infants

In general, the AAP and ACIP recommend that preterm and low-birth-weight infants be immunized at the usual chronologic age. Vaccine doses should not be altered based on the size of the infant. These recommendations apply to every vaccine except for hepatitis B vaccination. Studies have shown that the response to hepatitis B vaccine may be diminished in infants with birth weights less than 2000 g. Infants who weigh less than 2000 g at birth should have their initial hepatitis B vaccine delayed until they are 1 month of chronologic age. At this age, studies have shown that all preterm infants are as likely to respond to the vaccine as their full-term or larger counterparts. Preterm infants born to mothers who are HBsAg-positive or with unknown hepatitis B status should receive the vaccine and hepatitis B immunoglobulin within 12 hours of birth. This initial vaccine dose, however, should not be counted toward completion of the hepatitis B vaccine series, and 3 additional doses of hepatitis B should be given starting at 1 month chronologic age.[26]

Rotavirus Vaccine in Prematurity

Premature infants, who are at least 6 weeks of age, clinically stable, and being discharged from the hospital, can receive the rotavirus vaccine following the same guidelines as described in the rotavirus section.

Table 3
Contraindications and precautions of vaccines

Vaccine	Contraindication	Precaution
Hepatitis B	• Previous anaphylaxis	• Moderate or severe acute illness
DTaP	• Previous anaphylaxis • Encephalopathy within 7 d after DTaP	• Moderate or severe acute illness • History of arthus reaction following a prior dose of tetanus • Guillain-Barré syndrome within 6 wk after a tetanus toxoid–containing vaccine • Any of these events after a previous dose of DTaP: ○ Temperature of 105°F (40.5°C) or higher within 48 h ○ Continuous crying for 3 h or more within 48 h ○ Collapse or shocklike state within 48 h ○ Convulsion with or without fever within 3 d
TdaP	• Previous anaphylaxis • Encephalopathy within 7 d after DTaP	• Moderate or severe acute illness • History of arthus reaction following a prior dose of tetanus • Guillain-Barré syndrome within 6 wk after a tetanus toxoid–containing vaccine
IPV	• Previous anaphylaxis	• Moderate or severe acute illness • Pregnancy
HiB	• Previous anaphylaxis • Age less than 6 wk	• Moderate or severe acute illness
PCV	• Previous anaphylaxis	• Moderate or severe acute illness
Hepatitis A	• Previous anaphylaxis	• Moderate or severe acute illness • Pregnancy
Meningococcal	• Previous anaphylaxis	• Moderate or severe acute illness • History of Guillain-Barré syndrome (MCV4 only)
Varicella	• Previous anaphylaxis • Pregnancy • Children with high-dose immunosuppressive therapy • Children who are immunocompromised due to: ○ Malignancy ○ HIV/AIDS (although vaccination can be considered depending on CD4 counts (consult AAP Red Book)	• Moderate or severe acute illness • Administration of blood, plasma, and/or immune globulin within the past 11 mo

(*continued on next page*)

Table 3
(*continued*)

Vaccine	Contraindication	Precaution
MMR	• Previous anaphylaxis • Pregnancy • Severe Immunodeficiency defined as: ○ Hematologic and solid tumors ○ Congenital immunodeficiency ○ Long-term immunosuppressive therapy ○ Severely symptomatic HIV infection (HIV itself is not a contraindication)	• Moderate or severe acute illness • Administration of blood, plasma, and/or immune globulin within the past 11 mo • History of thrombocytopenia or thrombocytopenic purpura
Rotavirus	• Previous anaphylaxis • For latex allergic patients use Rotateq	• Moderate or severe acute illness • Moderate to severe acute gastroenteritis • Altered immunocompetence

Abbreviations: AAP, American Academy of Pediatrics; MCV4, quadrivalent meningococcal diphtheria vaccine; TdaP, tetanus, diphtheria, and pertussis (booster).

Data from Atkinson W, Wolfe S, Hamborsky J, editors. Centers for Disease Control and Prevention. Epidemiology and prevention of vaccine-preventable diseases. 12th edition. Washington, DC: Public Health Foundation; 2011.

Prevention of Respiratory Syncytial Virus with Palivizumab (Synagis)

Respiratory syncytial virus (RSV) causes acute respiratory tract illness in persons of all ages, and is the leading cause of bronchiolitis in children. Almost all children are infected by this virus by the age of 2 years, and the illness can be particularly severe, even fatal in certain risk groups. The factors associated with severe disease include gestation age less than 37 weeks, chronic pulmonary disease, congenital heart disease, immunodeficiency, neurologic disease, and congenital or anatomic defects of the airways.[27] Children with these specific risk factors are the targets for prevention of RSV using palivizumab.

Palivizumab is a humanized monoclonal antibody against RSV F glycoproteins, and is licensed for use in selected infants. The AAP recommends immunoprophylaxis with palivizumab for certain high-risk groups. Palivizumab is administered monthly at a dose of 15 mg/kg intramuscularly. The first dose is ideally administered 1 month before the start of the RSV season. The RSV season varies by geographic region, but in general usually lasts between November and April. Infants born during this season who meet the criteria for palivizumab are usually given their first dose before their hospital discharge.

The target group for children who should receive immunoprophylaxis against RSV includes infants with prematurity, bronchopulmonary dysplasia (BPD), and hemodynamically significant congenital heart disease. Based on the risks, benefits, and high cost of palivizumab, these recommendations were recently updated in 2009 to focus on infants at the highest risk of hospitalization from RSV. The new recommendations include risk factors to help decide whether certain groups should receive palivizumab. All children with BPD who have required medical therapy for their BPD within 6 months of the start of the RSV season, children with hemodynamically significant congenital heart disease, and infants should receive palivizumab regardless of risk factors.[7]

Table 4
Infants at high risk for hospitalization from RSV and who should be considered for palivizumab

Premature Infants	Additional Criteria
≤28 wk GA	≤12 mo of age at the start of RSV season
29–32 wk GA	≤6 mo of age at the start of RSV season
32–35 wk GA	≤6 mo of age at the start of RSV season, PLUS presence of risk factors (see below)
Risk Factors for 32–35 wk GA Infants	
School-age siblings	Low birth weight (<2500 g)
Daycare attendance	Multiple birth
Less than 12 wk at the start of RSV season	Family history of asthma or wheezing
Crowded living conditions	Congenital abnormalities of the airway
Exposure to tobacco smoke	Severe neuromuscular disease

Abbreviations: GA, gestational age; RSV, respiratory syncytial virus.

Infants who are born premature should also receive palivizumab depending on certain factors. The first is their gestational age and time of birth within the RSV season. For a summary of infants who should receive palivizumab based on gestational age and their age in reference to the RSV season, see **Table 4**.[28–30]

SUMMARY

Vaccination is a powerful and dynamic weapon in the clinician's arsenal in reducing the impact of infectious diseases in children. The field and schedules are constantly evolving, with significant changes resulting in new and exciting vaccines almost yearly. Special cases in pediatrics represent unique challenges and differences in vaccinations. Health care providers need to be knowledgable about the current vaccines and to remain up to date with the constant evolution. The CDC, ACIP, AAP, and ACOFP provide the latest recommendations, warnings, and news about vaccines and their use. It is important to constantly stay abreast of the ever-changing routine pediatric vaccination programs.

REFERENCES

1. Centers for Disease Control and Prevention (CDC). Progress toward elimination of *Haemophilus influenzae* type b invasive disease among infants and children—United States 1998-2000. MMWR Morb Mortal Wkly Rep 2002;51:234.
2. Johnson HL, Deloria-Knoll M, Levine OS, et al. Sustained reductions in invasive pneumococcal disease in the era of conjugate vaccine. J Infect Dis 2010;201:32.
3. US Department of Health and Human Services. Healthy people 2010 (conference ed., in 2 vols). Washington, DC: US Department of Health and Human Services; 2000. Available at: http://www.healthypeople.gov/2020/topicsobjectives2020/objectiveslist.aspx?topicid=23. Accessed March 17, 2011.
4. US Department of Health and Human Services. Healthy people 2020 (conference ed., in 2 vols). Washington, DC: US Department of Health and Human Services;

2010. Available at: http://www.healthypeople.gov/2020/topicsobjectives2020/objectiveslist.aspx?topicid=23. Accessed March 17, 2011.
5. Wilcox S, Koepke C, Levenson R, et al. Registry-driven, community based outreach: a randomized controlled trial. Am J Public Health 2001;91(9):1507–11.
6. Fiks AG, Hunter KF, Localio AR, et al. Impact of immunization at sick visits on well-child care. Pediatrics 2008;121(5):898–905.
7. Centers for Disease Control and Prevention. In: Atkinson W, Wolfe S, Hamborsky J, editors. Epidemiology and prevention of vaccine-preventable diseases. 12th edition. Washington, DC: Public Health Foundation; 2011. p. 345–6.
8. Schwartz B, Orenstein WA. Vaccination policies and programs: the federal government's role in making the system work. Prim Care 2001;28:697–711.
9. American Academy of Pediatrics. Hepatitis B. In: Pickering LK, editor. Red book: 2009 report of the Committee on Infectious Diseases. 28th edition. Elk Grove Village (IL): American Academy of Pediatrics; 2009. p. 10.
10. Lee C, Gong Y, Brok J, et al. Hepatitis B immunization for newborn infants of hepatitis B surface antigen positive mothers. Cochrane Database Syst Rev 2006;2:CD004790.
11. Hsu H, Shutt K, Moore MR, et al. Effect of pneumococcal conjugate vaccine on pneumococcal meningitis. N Engl J Med 2009;360:244–56.
12. Centers for Disease Control and Prevention (CDC). Licensure of a 13-valent pneumococcal Conjugate vaccine (PCV13) and recommendations for use among children—Advisory Committee on Immunization Practices (ACIP). MMWR Morb Mortal Wkly Rep 2010;59(9):258–61.
13. Committee on Infectious Disease. Recommended childhood and adolescent immunization schedules—United States, 2011. Pediatrics 2011;127:387.
14. Kim-Farley RJ, Bart KJ, Schonberger LB, et al. Poliomyelitis in the USA: virtual elimination of disease caused by wild virus. Lancet 1984;2(8415):1315.
15. Centers for Disease Control and Prevention (CDC). Updated recommendations of the Advisory Committee on Immunization Practices (ACIP) regarding routine poliovirus vaccination. MMWR Morb Mortal Wkly Rep 2009;58(30):829.
16. Peter G, Myers MG, National Vaccine Advisory Committee, National Vaccine Program Office. Intussusception, rotavirus, and oral vaccines: summary of a workshop. Pediatrics 2002;110(6):e67.
17. Dennehy PH, Goveia MG, Dallas MJ, et al. The integrated phase III safety profile of the pentavalent human-bovine (WC3) reassortant rotavirus vaccine. Int J Infect Dis 2007;11(Suppl 2):S36.
18. Centers for Disease Control and Prevention (CDC). Elimination of rubella and congenital rubella syndrome—United States, 1969-2004. MMWR Morb Mortal Wkly Rep 2005;54(11):279.
19. Offit PA. Evidence shows vaccines unrelated to autism. Immunization Action Coalition. Available at: www.immunize.org; http://www.immunize.org/catg.d/p4028.pdf. Accessed March 18, 2011.
20. Advisory Committee on Immunization Practices (ACIP), Fiore AE, Wasley A, et al. Prevention of hepatitis A through active or passive immunization: recommendations of the Advisory Committee on Immunization Practices (ACIP). MMWR Recomm Rep 2006;55(RR-7):1.
21. Granoff DM. Review of meningococcal group B vaccines. Clin Infect Dis 2010;50(Suppl 2):S54.
22. Centers for Disease Control and Prevention. Updated recommendations for use of meningococcal conjugate vaccines—Advisory Committee on Immunization Practices (ACIP), 2010. MMWR Morb Mortal Wkly Rep 2011;60(3):72–6.

23. Centers for Disease Control and Prevention. Preventing tetanus, diphtheria, and pertussis among adults: use of tetanus toxoid, reduced diphtheria toxoid and acellular pertussis vaccine. MMWR Morb Mortal Wkly Rep 2006;55(RR17):1–33.
24. Purdy KW, Hay JW, Botteman MF, et al. Evaluation of strategies for use of acellular pertussis vaccine in adolescents and adults: a cost-benefit analysis. Clin Infect Dis 2004;39(1):20.
25. Centers for Disease Control and Prevention (CDC). FDA licensure of bivalent human papillomavirus vaccine (HPV2, Cervarix) for use in females and updated HPV vaccination recommendations from the Advisory Committee on Immunization Practices (ACIP). MMWR Morb Mortal Wkly Rep 2010;59:626.
26. Markowitz LE, Dunnee EF, Saraiya M, et al. Quadrivalent human papillomavirus vaccine: recommendations of the Advisory Committee on Immunization Practices (ACIP). MMWR Recomm Rep 2007;56:1.
27. Centers for Disease Control and Prevention (CDC). FDA licensure of quadrivalent human papillomavirus vaccine (HPV4, Gardasil) for use in males and guidance from the Advisory Committee on Immunization Practices (ACIP). MMWR Morb Mortal Wkly Rep 2010;59:630.
28. Centers for Disease Control and Prevention. A comprehensive immunization strategy to eliminate transmission of hepatitis B virus infection in the United States. MMWR Recomm Rep 2005;54(RR-16):1–23.
29. Meissner HC. Selected populations at increased risk from respiratory syncytial virus infection. Pediatr Infect Dis J 2003;22(Suppl 2):S40.
30. Committee on Infectious Diseases. From the American Academy of Pediatrics: policy statements—modified recommendations for use of palivizumab for prevention of respiratory syncytial virus infections. Pediatrics 2009;124(6):1694.

Adult Vaccination

Christina M. Hillson, MD*, Joshua H. Barash, MD,
Edward M. Buchanan, MD

KEYWORDS

• Immunization • Vaccine • Adult

Immunization is one of the most clinically effective interventions available in modern medicine.[1] The success of immunization in the United States has been a major contributor to the increase in life expectancy and the decrease in infectious morbidities seen throughout the twentieth century.[2,3] This success story is largely attributed to the gains made in childhood immunization. Although adult vaccinations have the potential for similarly transforming benefits, lower vaccination rates in adults as compared with children have limited this effect.

Vaccination strategies in the adult population vary according to age, underlying medical conditions, lifestyle risks, and household contacts. For example, pneumococcal vaccination is recommended for all persons aged 65 years and older. It is also recommended for those with chronic pulmonary and cardiovascular disease as well as for those who smoke. Meningococcus vaccine is recommended not only for those with asplenia but also for young adults in high-density living situations. In these situations, vaccination is implemented to provide individuals with enhanced immunity and to protect others in the community via herd immunity.

In other situations, the primary goal of vaccination may be to protect the recipient's close contacts. For example, immunizing new parents against influenza and pertussis protects these individuals. More importantly, it reduces the likelihood of transmission to their newborn, who has a much greater morbidity and mortality risk from these diseases. This strategy, known as *cocooning*, applies to vaccinating close contacts of immunocompromised patients as well.

Over the past decade, the medical community has placed greater emphasis on educating health care providers and the public on the importance of adult vaccinations. The Centers for Disease Control and Prevention (CDC) began publishing an annual adult vaccination schedule in 2002, similar to the childhood schedule that has been published in various forms since 1983 (**Fig. 1**). In addition, Healthy People

Funding support: none.
Financial disclosures/conflicts of interest: the authors have nothing to disclose.
Thomas Jefferson University, Department of Family and Community Medicine, 833 Chestnut Street, Suite 301, Philadelphia, PA 19107, USA
* Corresponding author.
E-mail address: christina.hillson@jefferson.edu

Prim Care Clin Office Pract 38 (2011) 611–632
doi:10.1016/j.pop.2011.07.003 **primarycare.theclinics.com**
0095-4543/11/$ – see front matter

VACCINE ▼ AGE GROUP ▶	19–26 years	27–49 years	50–59 years	60–64 years	≥65 years
Influenza[1],*	1 dose annually				
Tetanus, diphtheria, pertussis (Td/Tdap)[2,*]	Substitute 1-time dose of Tdap for Td booster; then boost with Td every 10 years				Td booster every 10 years
Varicella[3,*]	2 doses				
Human papillomavirus (HPV)[4,*]	3 doses (females)				
Zoster[5]				1 dose	
Measles, mumps, rubella (MMR)[6,*]	1 or 2 doses		1 dose		
Pneumococcal (polysaccharide)[7,8]	1 or 2 doses				1 dose
Meningococcal[9,*]	1 or more doses				
Hepatitis A[10,*]	2 doses				
Hepatitis B[11,*]	3 doses				

*Covered by the Vaccine Injury Compensation Program

For all persons in this category who meet the age requirements and who lack evidence of immunity (e.g., lack documentation of vaccination or have no evidence of previous infection)

Recommended if some other risk factor is present (e.g., based on medical, occupational, lifestyle, or other indications)

No recommendation

Fig. 1. Recommended adult immunization schedule, by vaccine and age group. (*Courtesy of* the CDC and should be interpreted along with the corresponding footnotes. Available at: http://www.cdc.gov/vaccines/recs/schedules/downloads/adult/adult-schedule.pdf.)

2020 has set goals for adult vaccination rates against influenza, pneumococcus, zoster, and hepatitis B. These efforts reinforce the need for primary care physicians to provide appropriate vaccination throughout an individual's lifetime.

IMPROVING ADULT VACCINATION RATES

Despite the proved benefits of vaccines, adult immunization rates continue to be at unacceptably low levels. This is in contrast to the highly successful results of the pediatric vaccine delivery system. For example, coverage estimates for school entry vaccinations have consistently remained greater than 94% since 2003. In contrast, 2009 adult vaccination rates for influenza and pneumococcus range from 11% to 66% depending on the observed demographic risk group.[4–6] Consequently, 99% of the approximately 50,000 annual deaths from vaccine-preventable disease in the United States occur in adults.[1]

The causes for this discrepancy are numerous and readily observed by contrasting the pediatric and adult vaccination programs in the United States. The reasons can be broadly categorized into financial, public health oversight, and social/educational groupings.[7] From a financial perspective, pediatric vaccine costs are covered by a variety of mechanisms. Private insurance covers most recommended childhood vaccines. Uninsured children are covered through the federal Vaccines for Children Program and underinsured children through Section 317 of the Immunization Grant Program. Adults, however, are left without the Vaccines for Children Program safety net and have a lower priority than children for Section 317 funds. This leaves underinsured and uninsured individuals to pay for their own vaccinations, an obstacle that causes vaccination rates to plummet.

Public health oversight plays a greater role in childhood vaccination programs than for adults. School-based vaccination programs have entry requirements that act as a checkpoint to ensure children receive appropriate vaccines. In addition, childhood vaccination rates are closely monitored at the practice and community levels so that underimmunized populations can receive closer attention with walk-in clinics, school-based vaccinations, and so forth. Furthermore, electronic immunization registries allow multiple community immunization partners access to an individual's vaccination record to better coordinate care. Data from 2008 estimate that 75% of US children under age 6 are included in regional registries.[8]

Finally, public awareness of vaccinations for children is much greater than that for adults. As a result of strong public health campaigns, parents are aware of the expectation that from their first days of life, children begin a vaccination program in accordance with the national immunization program schedule. Well-child care visits are based on intervals recommended in this schedule. This contrasts with well-adult care, which competes for attention in practices where disease management plays a larger role than in pediatrics.

To improve adult vaccination rates, several recommendations targeted to individuals, providers, and public health initiatives have been proposed. Patient education through public service announcements and advertising can reach particular groups based on age, ethnicity, or demographic risks. Provider-based systems, such as vaccination reminders, standing orders, and outreach through convenient settings, are examples of proved strategies to improve vaccination rates. On a broader scale, increasing funding for uninsured and underinsured adults, creating adult immunization registries, and strengthening the CDC's ability to monitor adolescent and adult vaccination create an infrastructure to better enforce immunization for the entire population.[9,10]

ADULT VACCINATIONS

In addition to issues at the population level, unique challenges to adult vaccination exist at the provider level. Specifically, providers must consider age, occupation, lifestyle, and medical conditions to create an effective vaccination plan for an individual. Vaccines pertinent to the entire adult population include those against influenza and tetanus/diphtheria. Other vaccines are targeted to specific age groups, such as those against human papillomavirus (HPV), *Neisseria meningitidis, Streptococcus pneumoniae*, and herpes zoster. In some situations, vaccines may be warranted for an individual's risk of exposure to disease. These include hepatitis A, hepatitis B, and *N meningitidis.* Finally, certain individuals may have vaccine requirements due to exposure to susceptible populations. Pertussis, varicella, mumps, and rubella are included in this category.

This article reviews each of the vaccines in the adult immunization schedule and introduces immunization concepts pertinent to particular vaccines, such as primary and secondary vaccine failure, cocooning, and immune senescence.

Tetanus, Diphtheria, and Pertussis

Pertussis

Pathogenesis and clinical features *Bordetella pertussis* is a gram-negative coccobacillus that attacks respiratory epithelial cells. Classic pertussis is characterized by 3 phases. The catarrhal phase is the initial phase and consists of coryza, sneezing, and coughing. The coughing continues to worsen and after 1 to 2 weeks the paroxysmal stage ensues. This is characterized by bursts of rapid coughs that end with a long inspiratory effort accompanied by a high-pitched whoop. This lasts up to 6 weeks and is followed by the convalescent phase during which the cough gradually becomes less paroxysmal. The disease can be milder in older persons, but those who are infected may transmit it to unprotected infants. Older persons are often the source of infection for children.

Epidemiology Before the availability of the pertussis vaccine in the 1940s, more than 200,000 cases of pertussis were reported annually. Since widespread use of the vaccine began, incidence has decreased more than 80% compared with the prevaccine era. Despite decades of high vaccination coverage and the decreased incidence, pertussis has remained endemic and re-emerged as a public health problem in many countries in the past 2 decades. Waning of vaccine-induced immunity has been cited as one of the reasons for the observed epidemiologic trend.[11]

Diptheria

Pathogenesis and clinical features *Corynebacterium diphtheriae*, an aerobic gram-positive bacteria, produces a toxin that is responsible for local tissue destruction and membrane formation. Disease can involve almost any mucous membrane. The most common sites of infection are the pharynx and tonsils. Extensive membrane formation can result in respiratory obstruction and death.

Epidemiology Diphtheria was once a major cause of morbidity and mortality among children. A rapid decrease began with the widespread use of toxoid in the late 1940s. Most cases have occurred in unimmunized or inadequately immunized persons. Only 5 cases have been reported since 2000.

Tetanus

Pathogenesis and clinical features *Clostridium tetani*, a gram-positive, anaerobic rod, releases exotoxins that interfere with the release of neurotransmitters, leading to unopposed muscle contraction and spasm. *C tetani* usually enters the body through a wound. Trismus (lockjaw) appears early in its course, followed by neck stiffness, difficulty in swallowing, rigidity of abdominal muscles, and death.

Epidemiology In the late 1940s, tetanus toxoid was introduced into routine childhood immunization and tetanus incidence rates declined steadily. From 2000 through 2007 an average of 30 cases per year were reported. Almost all reported cases of tetanus are in persons who have either never been vaccinated or who completed a primary series but have not had a booster in the preceding 10 years.

Tetanus, diphtheria, and pertussis vaccine

Two products are licensed for use in the United States for adults up to 64 years old (Adacel and Boostrix). Both products contain tetanus toxoid, reduced diphtheria toxoid, and acellular pertussis vaccine (Tdap).

Immunogenicity and vaccine efficacy For both Tdap vaccines, the antibody response to a single dose of Tdap is similar to that after 3 doses of diphtheria toxoid, tetanus toxoid, and acellular pertussis vaccine (DTaP) in infants. These vaccines are assumed to have similar clinical efficacy as DTaP vaccine because a similar level of antibody to the components was achieved.

Vaccine highlights As discussed previously, waning immunity, also known as secondary vaccine failure, plays a critical role in the increased incidence of pertussis observed over the past 20 years. Immunity to pertussis wanes approximately 5 to 10 years after completion of childhood pertussis vaccination, leaving adolescents and adults susceptible.[12] In this age group, disease can vary from being asymptomatic to causing full disease. More importantly, infected individuals can transmit disease to newborns and infants under 1 year of age in whom morbidity and mortality rates are greatest. More than 50% of all newborn cases can be traced to an infectious family member. Furthermore, if parents of newborns are adequately immunized against pertussis, 35% to 55% of infant cases could be prevented.[13] This demonstrates the role of cocooning as a strategy to prevent neonatal pertussis.

To achieve this goal, the Advisory Committee on Immunization Practices (ACIP) recommends the following strategy in approaching Tdap vaccination for all adults with particular attention to those with exposure to newborns. At this time, data are not available to recommend for or against repeated Tdap booster throughout adulthood.

1. Adolescents and adults ages 11 to 64 years should receive a single dose of Tdap to replace tetanus and diphtheria toxoids vaccine (Td) for booster immunization against tetanus, diphtheria, and pertussis if they have not previously received Tdap.
2. Adults, including those 65 years and older, who have or who anticipate having close contact with an infant aged less than 12 months old should receive a single dose of Tdap to reduce the risk for transmitting pertussis.
3. When possible, women of childbearing age should receive Tdap before conception. The management of pregnant women who have never received Tdap vaccine is currently under revision. In May 2011, the ACIP proposed pregnant women be immunized after 20 weeks' gestation.[14] The CDC has not yet adopted these guidelines. Currently, CDC recommendations favor Tdap administration immediately postpartum except in outbreak situations.
4. Health care personnel who work in hospitals or ambulatory care settings and have direct patient contact should receive a single dose of Tdap as soon as feasible if they have not previously received Tdap.

5. Adults with uncertain histories of a complete primary vaccination series with diphtheria and tetanus toxoid–containing vaccines should begin or complete a primary vaccination series: Tdap is the preferred first dose, followed by Td 4 weeks later, and the third Td dose 6 to 12 months after the second.

Adults as listed previously, Tdap can be administered regardless of the interval since the last tetanus toxoid–containing vaccine or diphtheria toxoid–containing vaccine.

Streptococcous Pneumoniae

Pathogenesis and clinical features

S pneumoniae is a gram-positive, anaerobic organism, which inhabits the respiratory tract and may be isolated from the nasopharynx of 5% to 70% of healthy adults. Transmission occurs via respiratory droplets. The major clinical diseases caused by pneumococcus are pneumonia, bacteremia, and meningitis.

Epidemiology

More than 40,000 cases and more than 4400 deaths from invasive pneumococcal disease (bacteremia and meningitis) are estimated to have occurred in the United States in 2007. More than half of these cases occurred in adults who had an indication for pneumococcal vaccination. Healthy People 2020 calls for high-risk persons ages 18 to 64 years and persons 65 years and older to reach immunization rates of 60% and 90%, respectively, by 2020. In 2008, these rates were 17% and 60%, respectively. There is much work to be done to improve these immunization rates.[15]

Pneumococcal vaccine

Pneumococcal polysaccharide vaccine (PPSV) is composed of purified preparations of pneumococcal capsular polysaccharide. The first polysaccharide pneumococcal vaccine was licensed in the United States in 1977. Pneumovax, a 23-valent polysaccharide vaccine, is the current (PPSV23) available in the United States.

Immunogenicity and vaccine effectiveness More than 80% of healthy adults who receive PPSV23 develop antibodies against the serotypes contained in the vaccine. Elevated antibody levels persist for at least 5 years in healthy adults but decline more quickly in persons with certain underlying illnesses. Overall, the vaccine is 60% to 70% effective in preventing invasive disease. Although the vaccine may not be as effective in some persons, especially those who are immunosuppressed, it is still recommended for such persons because they are at high risk of developing severe disease.

Vaccine highlights The pneumococcal vaccine should be administered once to all adults 65 years of age and older. The vaccine is also indicated for persons 19 to 64 years, with any of the underlying medical conditions listed in **Fig. 2**.

In 2008, ACIP added asthma and smoking as indications PPSV for adults 19 years of age and older. These groups demonstrate increased risk of invasive pneumococcal disease. Healthy adults age 18 to 64 years who smoke are 4 times as likely to develop invasive pneumococcal disease than their nonsmoking counterparts (odds ratio [OR] 4.1; 95% CI, 2.4–7.3).[16] Persons with asthma are twice as likely to suffer from invasive pneumococcal disease compared with those without asthma (OR 2.4; 95% CI, 1.9–3.1).[17]

Revaccination with PPSV is not generally recommended. It is indicated, however, one time after 5 years for persons 19 to 64 years old with functional or anatomic asplenia and for persons with immunocompromising conditions. Those adults who received PPSV before age 65 years for any indication should receive another dose of the

INDICATION ▶ / VACCINE ▼	Pregnancy	Immunocompromising conditions (excluding human immunodeficiency virus [HIV])[3,5,6,13]	HIV infection[3,6,12,13] CD4+ T lymphocyte count		Diabetes, heart disease, chronic lung disease, chronic alcoholism	Asplenia[12] (including elective splenectomy) and persistent complement component deficiencies	Chronic liver disease	Kidney failure, end-stage renal disease, receipt of hemodialysis	Health-care personnel
			<200 cells/μL	≥200 cells/μL					
Influenza[1,*]					1 dose TIV annually				1 dose TIV or LAIV annually
Tetanus, diphtheria, pertussis (Td/Tdap)[2,*]	Td					Substitute 1-time dose of Tdap for Td booster; then boost with Td every 10 years			
Varicella[3,*]		Contraindicated				2 doses			
Human papillomavirus (HPV)[4,*]					3 doses through age 26 years				
Zoster[5]		Contraindicated					1 dose		
Measles, mumps, rubella[6,*]		Contraindicated				1 or 2 doses			
Pneumococcal (polysaccharide)[7,8]					1 or 2 doses				
Meningococcal[9,*]			1 or more doses						
Hepatitis A[10,*]				2 doses					
Hepatitis B[11,*]						3 doses			

*Covered by the Vaccine Injury Compensation Program

[Light shading] For all persons in this category who meet the age requirements and who lack evidence of immunity (e.g., lack documentation of vaccination or have no evidence of previous infection)

[Dark shading] Recommended if some other risk factor is present (e.g., on the basis of medical, occupational, lifestyle, or other indications)

[White] No recommendation

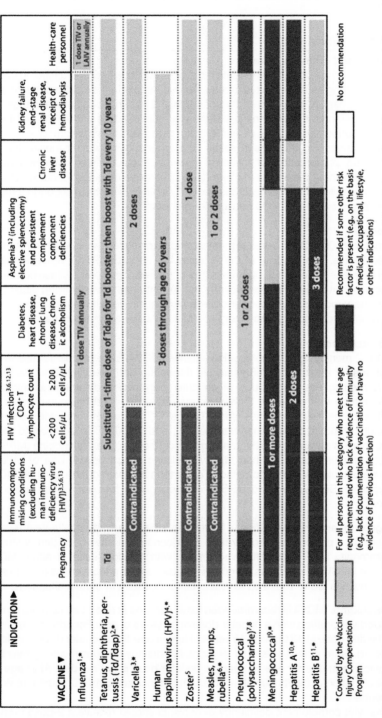

Fig. 2. Vaccines that might be indicated for adults based on medical and other indications. (*Courtesy of* the CDC and should be interpreted along with the corresponding footnotes. Available at: http://www.cdc.gov/vaccines/recs/schedules/downloads/adult/adult-schedule.pdf.)

vaccine at age 65 years or later if at least 5 years have passed since their previous dose.[18,19]

Neisseria Meningitidis

Pathogenesis and clinical features

N meningitidis, an aerobic, gram-negative diplococcus, has become a leading cause of bacterial meningitis in the United States. Aerosol respiratory droplets or secretions from the nasopharynx of colonized persons transmit meningococci. In less than 1% of colonized persons, the bacteria penetrate the mucosal cells and enter the bloodstream. In approximately 50% of bacteremic persons, the organism crosses the blood-brain barrier into the cerebrospinal fluid and causes purulent meningitis, the most common presentation of invasive meningococcal disease. Meningococcal sepsis occurs without meningitis in 5% to 20% of invasive meningococcal infections. The communicability of *N meningitidis* is generally limited. The risk of secondary transmission is 2 to 4 cases per 1000 household members.[20]

Epidemiology

Approximately 1000 to 3000 cases of meningococcal disease are reported each year in the United States. The majority of these cases are sporadic (95%); however, since 1991, the frequency of localized outbreaks has increased.[21] Invasive disease outbreaks are associated with young adults recently moving into high-density living situations, such as military recruits and first-year college students in dormitories. The proportion of cases among adolescents and young adults has increased in recent years.

Meningococcal vaccine

As of 2011, 2 meningococcal conjugate vaccines (MCV4) are available for use in the United States for adults up to 55 years old (Menactra and Menveo). Both vaccines contain *N meningiditis* serogroups of capsular polysaccharide antigens linked to a protein epitope that evokes a T-cell immune response. Three main serotypes are responsible for the majority of disease: B, C, and Y. The current conjugate quadrivalent vaccines contain polysaccharides A, C, Y, and W-135.[20] In addition to these vaccines, there is an unconjugated meningococcal polysaccharide vaccine (MPSV4) that is less immunogenic and has rapidly declining effectiveness. Use of MPSV4 (Menomune) should be limited to persons older than 55 years of age or when MCV4 is not available. Both MCV4 and MPSV4 are acceptable for use in meningococcal outbreaks.[20]

Immunogenicity and vaccine efficacy More than 98% of healthy adults who receive MCV4 develop a protective antibody titer. Postlicensure studies have demonstrated waning immunity by 5 years after vaccination with a single dose of either MCV4 vaccine. The MPSV4 vaccine has demonstrated decreased effectiveness after 3 years in adults. This has led to the need for vaccination boosters in certain situations.

Vaccine highlights MCV4 is recommended for all persons at age 11 or 12 years as part of childhood vaccination with a booster dose at 16 years of age. For adolescents who receive the first dose at 13 through 15 years of age, a one-time booster dose should be administered, preferably at age 16 to 18 years. For healthy persons receiving their first dose of vaccine at or after age 16 years, a booster dose is not needed. After age 21, routine vaccination of healthy adults who are not at increased risk for exposure is not recommended.

Persons with complement deficiency or asplenia should receive a 2-dose primary series administered 8 weeks apart and receive subsequent booster doses every 5 years through age 55. If one dose has already been administered, then a booster dose should be given at the earliest opportunity, with subsequent booster doses every 5 years through age 55 (see **Fig. 2** for additional indications).

Human Papillomavirus

Pathogenesis and clinical features

HPV, a small, double-stranded DNA virus, infects basal epithelium. More than 100 HPV types have been identified, most of which infect the cutaneous epithelium and cause common skin warts. Other strains infect cervical epithelium and can cause cervical dysplasia and cervical cancer. Persistent infection with a high-risk type is the most significant risk factor for the development of cervical cancer and is considered a necessary precursor to this disease.[22] High-risk HPV types are detected in 99% of cervical cancers. Together, HPV types 16 and 18 are responsible for 70% of cervical neoplasia both in the United States and worldwide.

HPV also plays a role in the development squamous carcinoma of the anus, vagina, vulva, and oral cavity as well as that of genital warts. It is associated with approximately 90% of anal cancer, 40% of penile cancer, 60% of vaginal cancer, 50% of vulvar cancers, 25% of oral cavity cancers, and 35% of oropharyngeal cancers.[23]

Epidemiology

Transmission occurs most frequently with genital contact. Nonsexual routes of HPV transmission are rare but include transmission from a woman to a newborn infant at the time of birth. Risk factors for HPV infection are related to sexual behavior, including the number of sex partners, lifetime history of sex partners, and partners' sexual history.

HPV vaccine

As of 2011, 2 HPV vaccines are licensed for use in the United States, a bivalent vaccine (Cervarix), which is protective against HPV types 16 and 18, and a quadrivalent vaccine (Gardasil) that protects against HPV types 6, 11, 16, and 18.

Immunogenicity and vaccine efficacy In studies conducted to date, more than 99.5% of participants receiving quadrivalent vaccine developed an antibody response to all 4 HPV types in the vaccine 1 month after completing the 3-dose series. The clinical efficacy against cervical disease in women administered the vaccine from ages 14 to 26 years is 100% for the prevention of HPV type 16–related or HPV type 18–related cervical intraepithelial neoplasia (CIN) 2/3 or adenocarcinoma in situ. Efficacy against any CIN due to HPV types 6, 11, 16, or 18 was 95%. The quadrivalent vaccine is 99% effective in preventing genital warts related to HPV types 6 and 11. More than 90% of genital warts are caused by HPV types 6 and 11.[24]

The majority of these studies were conducted on women less than 27 years of age. More recently, in 2011, the FUTURE III trial evaluated the quadrivalent HPV vaccine in a placebo-controlled, double-blind, randomized study of more than 3000 women ages 24 to 45 years. The primary analysis followed women who were naive to HPV types 6, 11, 16, and 18 and who received all 3 vaccinations within 1 year. The efficacy of the vaccine against HPV types 6–, 11–, 16–, or 18–related persistent infection; genital warts; vulvar and vaginal lesions; and CIN of any grade was 88.7% (95% CI, 78.1–94.8).[25] Although not as effective as for women under 27 years old, there is a benefit for women up to age 45. As a result, in 2011 Canada extended the use of the quadrivalent vaccine in women up to age 45. In the United States, however, the Food and Drug Administration (FDA) has not endorsed its use in women over age 26.

The HPV vaccine has also been shown to be immunogenic and safe in men. The vaccine is 85.6% effective at preventing persistent infection with HPV types 6, 11,

16, and 18 in men who are vaccinated before HPV exposure with these types and 90.4% effective at preventing anogenital lesions related to these types.[26]

Vaccine highlights The ACIP recommends starting the HPV vaccine series in girls at ages 11 to 12 years, but it may be given as early as 9 years of age. Catch-up vaccination is recommended for girls and women 13 through 26 years of age who have not been previously vaccinated or who have not completed the full series. In 2009, the FDA approved the quadrivalent HPV vaccine for men ages 9 through 26 to reduce their likelihood of acquiring genital warts. In 2010, the FDA approved the quadrivalent vaccine for the prevention of anal cancer caused by HPV types 16 and 18 and for the prevention of anal intraepithelial neoplasia (AIN) grades 1, 2, and 3 (anal dysplasias and precancerous lesions) caused by HPV types 6, 11, 16, and 18, in males and females 9 through 26 years of age.[22] Currently there are not enough data to recommend the HPV vaccine for the prevention of oropharyngeal cancers.[27]

HPV vaccines are most effective when given before exposure to HPV through sexual contact; however, individuals who may have already been exposed to HPV should still be vaccinated. When feasible, the same type of vaccination should be used throughout the series. If it is not available or the type of vaccine used at initiation is unknown, however, this should not be a barrier to vaccination and no changes need to be made to the dosing schedule. The duration of protection from HPV vaccine is not known. Studies to investigate this issue are in progress. Booster doses are not recommended at this time.

Hepatitis A

Pathogenesis and clinical features

The hepatitis A virus (HAV) is an RNA virus belonging to the picornavirus family. It is transmitted primarily through the fecal-oral route. The infection caused by the HAV can either be asymptomatic or symptomatic. Although hepatitis A infection is usually self-limiting without serious sequelae, it can cause considerable morbidity.

Epidemiology

Within the Unites States, hepatitis A has historically caused large outbreaks every 10 years. Rates have continued to fall to all-time lows, however, since 1995. The use of the vaccine, released in 1995, is likely contributing to these declining rates.[28] In 2007, the incidence of hepatitis A was the lowest ever reported.[29]

Hepatitis A vaccine

The vaccine is an inactivated whole virus vaccine that was developed in 1995. Currently 2 forms are available (havrix and Vaqta). The vaccine also comes in a combination form with hepatitis B (Twinrix).

Immunogenicity and vaccine efficacy The success of the vaccine is evident by the significant decrease in acute hepatitis A infection since its debut, with a 92% decline in incidence rate in the past decade.[30] Immunogenicity studies reveal close to a 100% seroconversion rate after primary vaccination in adults.[28] The estimated duration of adequate antibody levels is between 20 and 30 years after vaccination.

Vaccine highlights The introduction of hepatitis A vaccine into the national immunization program commenced in a stepwise fashion. In 1996, the ACIP recommended vaccinating travelers and at-risk populations. This had little national effect, so in 1999 the recommendations were expanded to include children 2 years or older living in high-incidence areas. This had a significant impact and decreased the incidence among children by 87%.[29] Finally, in 2006, the ACIP expanded its recommendations to all children 1 year of age or older in addition to certain adult groups.

Adults at-risk for complications from HAV infection and those in high-risk populations should be vaccinated. These include injection-drug users, men who have sex with men, those with a close personal contact with an international adoptee from a country of high/intermediate endemicity[1] during the first 60 days of arrival, persons with occupational exposure to hepatitis A, those receiving clotting factor concentrate, and persons traveling to countries with high/intermediate endemicity[1] (see **Fig. 2** for additional indications).

Hepatitis B

Pathogenesis and clinical features

The hepatitis B virus (HBV) is a DNA virus that is part of the Hepadnaviridae family. It is transmitted through mucosal or percutaneous exposure to infected blood and bodily fluids, specifically serum, semen, and saliva. Less than 50% of adults show initial signs and symptoms. Acute infection ranges from asymptomatic or mild disease to, in rare cases, fulminant hepatitis.[31]

The majority of HBV-related morbidity and mortality comes from chronic hepatitis B infection, which can result in cirrhosis, liver cancer, and/or liver failure. Nationally, an estimated 4000 adults die annually from hepatitis B–related cirrhosis, and 1500 die from hepatitis B–related liver cancer. The risk of chronic hepatitis B infection decreases with age; approximately 95% of adults recover completely from HBV infection and do not become chronically infected, whereas 80% and 90% of infants infected perinatally develop chronic infection.[32]

Epidemiology

The incidence of hepatitis B hit an all-time high in the United States during the mid-1980s with more than 25,000 cases reported per year. Since that time, the number of cases has significantly declined. In 2007, only 4519 cases of acute hepatitis B in the United States were reported. Rates are highest among adults, in particular men ages 25 to 44 years, and approximately 79% of persons with newly acquired hepatitis B are known to engage in high-risk sexual behaviors or injection drug use.[31]

Hepatitis B vaccine

The hepatitis B vaccine has been used in the United States since 1986, when it was recommended for high-risk individuals. Starting in 1991, vaccination has been recommended for all infants. In 2005, the ACIP established a comprehensive 4-pronged strategy to eliminate HBV transmission, which includes vaccination of high-risk adults.

High-risk adults needing the vaccine include household contacts and sex partners of hepatitis B surface antigen–positive people, intravenous drug users, sexually active individuals not in a long-term monogamous relationship (>1 sexual partner/6 months), men who have sex with men, persons seeking sexually transmitted disease evaluation and/or treatment, and international travelers to regions with high or intermediate levels of endemic HBV infection[31] (see **Fig. 2** for additional indications).

Immunogenicity and vaccine efficacy The vaccine has an efficacy of greater than 90% and is effective against all subtypes. Since 1991, when a national strategy to eliminate HBV infection was implemented in the United States, the incidence of reported acute hepatitis B has declined 78%.[32]

---

[1] For a list of endemic areas, see: http://wwwnc.cdc.gov/travel/content/diseases.aspx.

Vaccine highlights A challenge to vaccination is that 5% to 10% of individuals do not respond to the current vaccines (primary vaccine failure). Medically healthy nonresponders should receive 1 or more additional doses.[31] Up to 50% of nonresponders mount a response after 3 additional doses, so an acceptable option is to repeat the entire series.[31] More studies need to be performed to determine optimal follow-up for at-risk individuals.

Primary Varicella Infection (Chickenpox)

Pathogenesis and clinical features

The varicella zoster virus (VZV) is a member of the herpesvirus family of DNA viruses. Varicella is highly infectious, with up to a 90% secondary attack rate in nonimmunized individuals. VZV is transmitted by direct contact, either by inhalation of aerosols from vesicular fluid or aerosolized respiratory tract secretions. The illness usually starts with a mild viral prodrome followed by a rash. The rash is generalized and pruritic and progresses rapidly from macules to papules to vesicular lesions before crusting. A person is considered infectious 1 to 2 days before the onset of the rash and until all lesions are encrusted.[33]

Epidemiology

Prior to the development of the vaccine, varicella was endemic in the United States and almost all persons acquired the infection by adulthood. There were an estimated 4 million cases per year, with adults accounting for 7% of these cases. Since the development of the vaccine, varicella cases have declined by 83% to 93%.[34]

Varicella vaccine

A vaccine for VZV prevention was first introduced in 1995. At present there are 2 varicella-containing vaccines for the prevention of primary infection: varicella vaccine (Varivax) and a combination measles-mumps-rubella-varicella (MMRV) vaccine (ProQuad).

Immunogenicity and vaccine effectiveness Approximately 78% of adults develop an antibody response after 1 dose, and 99% develop an adequate response after a second dose given 4 to 8 weeks later. Immunity seems to be long lasting and is thought to be permanent in the majority of vaccinated individuals.[34]

Vaccine highlights Routine vaccination is recommended for all healthy nonpregnant adults without evidence of immunity (see **Table 1** for immunity criteria). Pregnant women who become infected with VZV are at risk for transmission of the virus to their children, which can cause congenital defects as well as neonatal varicella and other complications. Therefore, women who present for preconception counseling should be assessed for immunity to varicella. If a woman is found to be nonimmune, she should be vaccinated. As with any live attenuated vaccine, a woman should not become pregnant until 4 weeks after immunization. No studies to date, however, have found the vaccine harmful to the fetus and the risk remains theoretic. Therefore, if the vaccine is given during pregnancy, it is not an indication for termination. Because the vaccine is not recommended during pregnancy, women of childbearing age should be screened for pregnancy before vaccination.

Herpes Zoster (Shingles)

Pathogenesis and clinical features

Zoster is a localized, generally painful cutaneous eruption that occurs most frequently among older adults and immunocompromised persons. It is caused by reactivation of latent varicella zoster virus, persisting latently in the dorsal root ganglia. A common complication of zoster is postherpetic neuralgia, a chronic, often debilitating pain condition that can last months or even years. Other complications can include zoster opthalmicus (eye involvement) and Ramsay Hunt syndrome (peripheral facial nerve palsy), among others.[35]

Epidemiology

Approximately 1 in 3 persons develops zoster during a lifetime, resulting in an estimated 1 million episodes in the United States annually. The risk for postherpetic neuralgia in patients with zoster is 10% to 18%.[36]

Herpes zoster vaccine

In May 2006, a vaccine containing a live, attenuated strain of VZV was developed to prevent zoster (Zostavax). The zoster vaccine is recommended for all persons aged 60 years and older. The vaccine can be given to persons who have had a previous episode of zoster or who have chronic medical conditions.

Vaccine immunogenicity and efficacy In a large, randomized, clinical trial of persons 60 years or older, the zoster vaccine was effective at preventing zoster in 51% of cases. In those that developed Zoster, the vaccine reduced the severity and duration of pain by 57% and prevented postherpetic neuralgia in approximately 66% of cases.[36] The duration of the protective effects of herpes zoster vaccine has not been determined; current studies show that protection lasts at least 4 years. Efficacy of the vaccine decreases with age, with it most effective in the 60-year-old to 69-year-old age group versus those 70 years and older.

Influenza

Pathogenesis and clinical features

Influenza is a contagious respiratory illness. Symptoms can include fever, cough, headache, fatigue, body aches, coryza, and vomiting or diarrhea. In the general population, it is usually a self-limited infection; however, it is associated with increased morbidity and mortality in certain high-risk populations. Transmission occurs through person-to-person contact with respiratory droplets.

Influenza A and B are the 2 types of influenza viruses that cause epidemic human disease worldwide. Influenza A viruses are further categorized into subtypes based on their surface antigens (hemagglutinin and neuraminidase). New influenza virus variants result from genetic mutations that alter these antigenic proteins. When a more significant change occurs, termed *antigenic shift*, a subtype has the potential to cause a pandemic.

Epidemiology

During annual epidemics, rates of serious illness and death are highest among persons aged 65 years and older, children ages less than 2 years, and persons of any age who have at-risk medical conditions. Influenza epidemics were associated with estimated annual averages of approximately 36,000 deaths between 1990 and 1999 and approximately 226,000 hospitalizations between 1979 and 2001.[37]

Influenza vaccine

Because the influenza virus has a high mutation rate, it compromises the ability of the immune system to protect against new variants each season. Therefore, new vaccine is produced annually to match the predicted predominant strain for the coming year. There are 2 forms of the influenza vaccine, an inactivated trivalent intramuscular influenza vaccine (TIV) and a trivalent live attenuated influenza vaccine (LAIV) form that is

Table 1
Vaccine contraindications and precautions

Vaccine	Contraindications	Precautions
Tdap	Severe allergic reaction (eg, anaphylaxis) after a previous dose or to a vaccine component Encephalopathy (eg, coma, decreased level of consciousness, prolonged seizures) not attributable to another identifiable cause within 7 days of administration of previous dose of DTP or DTaP	Guillian-Barré syndrome (GBS) within 6 wk after a previous dose of tetanus toxoid–containing vaccine Progressive or unstable neurologic disorder, uncontrolled seizures, or progressive encephalopathy: defer vaccination until a treatment regimen has been established and the condition has stabilized History of arthus-type hypersensitivity reactions after a previous dose of tetanus toxoid–containing vaccine: defer vaccination until at least 10 years have elapsed since the last tetanus toxoid–containing vaccine Moderate or severe acute illness with or without fever
Dt, Td	Severe allergic reaction (eg, anaphylaxis) after a previous dose or to a vaccine component	GBS within 6 wk after previous dose of tetanus toxoid–containing vaccine History of arthus-type hypersensitivity reactions after a previous dose of tetanus toxoid–containing vaccine: defer vaccination until at least 10 years have elapsed since the last tetanus toxoid–containing vaccine Moderate or severe acute illness with or without fever
Pneumococcal	Severe allergic reaction (eg, anaphylaxis) after a previous dose (of PCV7, PCV13, or any diphtheria toxoid–containing vaccine) or to a component of a vaccine	Moderate or severe acute illness with or without fever

Hepatitis B	Severe allergic reaction (eg, anaphylaxis) after previous dose or to a vaccine component	Moderate or severe acute illness with or without fever
Hepatitis A	Severe allergic reaction (eg, anaphylaxis) after a previous dose or to a vaccine component	Pregnancy Moderate or severe acute illness with or without fever
MMR	Severe allergic reaction (eg, anaphylaxis) after a previous dose or to a vaccine component Pregnancy Known severe immunodeficiency (eg, from hematologic and solid tumors, receipt of chemotherapy, congenital immunodeficiency, long-term immunosuppressive therapy (2 wk of 20 mg/d prednisone); or patients with HIV infection who are severely immunocompromised)	Pregnancy Moderate or severe acute illness with or without fever Recent (within 11 months) receipt of antibody-containing blood product (specific interval depends on product) History of thrombocytopenia or thrombocytopenic purpura Need for tuberculin skin testing Moderate or severe acute illness with or without fever
Varicella	Severe allergic reaction (eg, anaphylaxis) after a previous dose or to a vaccine component Known severe immunodeficiency (eg, from hematologic and solid tumors, receipt of chemotherapy, congenital immunodeficiency, long-term immunosuppressive therapy4; or patients with HIV infection who are severely immunocompromised)3 Pregnancy	Recent (within 11 months) receipt of antibody-containing blood product (specific interval depends on product)8 Moderate or severe acute illness with or without fever
Zoster	Severe allergic reaction (eg, anaphylaxis) after a previous dose or to a vaccine component	Moderate or severe acute illness with or without fever

(*continued on next page*)

Table 1
(*continued*)

Vaccine	Contraindications	Precautions
	Substantial suppression of cellular immunity Pregnancy	
Influenza (TIV)	Severe allergic reaction (eg, anaphylaxis) after a previous dose or to a vaccine component, including egg protein	GBS within 6 wk of previous dose of influenza vaccine Moderate or severe acute illness with or without fever
Influenza (LAIV)	Severe allergic reaction (eg, anaphylaxis) after a previous dose or to a vaccine component, including egg protein Pregnancy Immunosuppression Medical conditions: asthma, pulmonary or cardiovascular disease (except isolated hypertension); renal, hepatic, neurologic, neuromuscular, hematologic or metabolic disorders	GBS within 6 wk of previous dose of influenza vaccine Moderate or severe acute illness with or without fever
HPV	Severe allergic reaction (eg, anaphylaxis) after a previous dose or to a vaccine component	Pregnancy Moderate or severe acute illness with or without fever
Meningococcal	Severe allergic reaction (eg, anaphylaxis) after a previous dose or to a vaccine component	Moderate or severe acute illness with or without fever

Abbreviations: Dt, diptheria-tetanus toxoid; PCV, pneumococcal conjugate vaccine.
Courtesy of the CDC. Available at: http://www.cdc.gov/vaccines/recs/vac-admin/contraindications-vacc.htm.

delivered via intranasal spray. The TIV form is approved for all adults, whereas the LAIV vaccine is approved for nonpregnant individuals, ages 2 to 49 years. LAIV is contraindicated in adults with certain medical conditions (**Box 1**).

Immunogenicity and vaccine efficacy The efficacy of influenza vaccines depends on the age and immunocompetence of the vaccine recipient as well as the degree of similarity between the vaccine and the circulating virus. Studies conducted during years when the vaccine and circulating viruses are antigenically similar reveal that TIV is 70% to 90% effective in preventing illness in healthy adults.[38] Efficacy or effectiveness against influenza was substantially lower in studies conducted during influenza seasons when the vaccine strains were antigenically dissimilar to the majority of circulating strains. Both LAIV and TIV contain strains of influenza viruses that are equivalent antigenically to the annually recommended 3 strains: 1 influenza A virus subtype H3N2, 1 influenza A virus subtype H1N1, and 1 influenza B virus.

Vaccine highlights All individuals 6 months of age and older should receive the influenza vaccine. This includes all adults and pregnant women. The vaccine has been proved safe and beneficial in pregnancy. Studies show that vaccinating pregnant women results in a 29% reduction in febrile respiratory illness and an even greater reduction of 36% in their infants in the first 6 months of life.[39]

In an effort to decrease barriers to influenza vaccination, the ACIP in 2011 recommended that a history of allergy to eggs be changed from a contraindication to a precaution for influenza vaccination. This recommendation is specifically for the inactivated (TIV) form of the influenza vaccine. An anaphylactic reaction to eggs

Box 1
Evidence of immunity to varicella

Evidence of immunity to varicella includes any of the following:

- Documentation of age-appropriate vaccination with a varicella vaccine
  - Preschool-aged children (ie, aged >12 months): 1 dose
  - School-aged children, adolescents, and adults: 2 doses[a]
- Laboratory evidence of immunity[b] or laboratory confirmation of disease
- Birth in the United States before 1980[c]
- Diagnosis or verification of a history of varicella disease by a health care provider[d]
- Diagnosis or verification of a history of herpes zoster by a health care provider

[a] For children who received their first dose at age <13 years and for whom the interval between the 2 doses was >28 days, the second dose is considered valid.
[b] Commercial assays can be used to assess disease-induced immunity, but they lack sensitivity to always detect vaccine-induced immunity (ie, they might yield false-negative results).
[c] For health care personnel, pregnant women, and immunocompromised persons, birth before 1980 should not be considered evidence of immunity.
[d] Verification of history or diagnosis of typical disease can be provided by any health care provider (eg, school or occupational clinic nurse, nurse practitioner, physician assistant, or physician). For persons reporting a history of, or reporting with, atypical or mild cases, assessment by a physician or their designee is recommended, and one of the following should be sought: (1) an epidemiologic link to a typical varicella case to a laboratory-confirmed case or (2) evidence of laboratory confirmation, if it was performed at the time of acute disease. When such documentation is lacking, persons should not be considered as having a valid history of disease because other diseases might mimic mild atypical varicella.

Courtesy of CDC. Available at: http://www.cdc.gov/mmwr/preview/mmwrhtml/rr5604a1.htm.

remains a contraindication to use. For patients with a history of egg allergy without anaphylaxis, there is no need to divide doses or perform skin testing before vaccination, but they should be observed for 30 minutes after vaccination.[14]

Deterioration of the immune system accompanies aging, a multifactorial condition termed, *immunosenescence*.[40] Older individuals have a decreased ability to respond to infection and a decreased ability to mount an immune response to vaccinations. To compensate for this decreased immune response, adults 65 years of age and older may receive either the standard TIV dose or a higher-dose version of the influenza vaccine, which contains 4 times the amount of antigen. A higher antibody level has been seen in response to this vaccination, but it is not yet clear if the vaccine will clinically decrease influenza disease in this population.[33]

Measles, Mumps, Rubella

Measles

Pathogenesis and clinical features Measles is a paramyxovirius spread by respiratory transmission with initial infection occurring in the nasopharynx. This is followed by a 2-staged viremia first attacking the lymphatic system, then involving the respiratory tract and other organs. With an incubation period of 10 to 12 days, measles manifests with high fevers followed by the classic triad of cough, coryza, and conjunctivitis. The presence of Koplik spots (white exanthem of mucosal surfaces) and a maculopapular rash starting at the hairline and progressing caudally to involve the entire body then follow. Complications of the disease include encephalitis and pneumonia.[41]

Epidemiology At the start of the twenty-first century, measles was the leading cause of vaccine-preventable death in children worldwide.[42] Due to a successful immunization program, endemic spread has been eliminated in the United States. Sporadic outbreaks, however, continue to be imported from other nations and spread in communities with low vaccination rates. Measles is one of the first vaccine-preventable diseases to reappear once vaccination rates drop and herd immunity is lost. In the United Kingdom, where measles vaccination coverage has dropped to 85%, the disease is once again endemic.[43]

Mumps

Pathogenesis and clinical features Mumps virus is a paramyxovirus also spread by respiratory transmission with reproduction in the nasopharynx. Generalized viremia then allows for spread to other organs, such as the meninges and glands, including the parotids and testes. The incubation period is 16 to 18 days with a nonspecific prodromal period. The most common clinical manifestation is parotitis occurring in up to 40% of patients. The remaining 60% of infected individuals, however, may be asymptomatic or have nonspecific manifestations of disease. The most common complication of mumps infection in adults is orchitis, occurring in 37% of men. This can result in testicular atrophy although infertility is uncommon. Aseptic meningitis occurs in up to 62% of patients although this is symptomatic in only 15% of cases. In addition, acute, permanent hearing loss occurs in 1 per 20,000 cases.[44]

Epidemiology Mumps was once a common cause of aseptic meningitis and sensorineural hearing loss in the prevaccine era. Since the introduction of live vaccine in 1967, reported cases dropped precipitously from an estimated 160,000 cases per year to a low of 231 cases in 2003. Two outbreaks have occurred in the past 5 years, the most serious of which was in 2006 when 6584 cases were reported, most commonly affecting college students. Both outbreaks seem to be linked to outbreaks in the United Kingdom although the majority of occurrences in the United States have been in immunized individuals.[45] The limited spread of these outbreaks emphasizes the importance of herd immunity in controlling this disease.

Rubella

Pathogenesis and clinical features Rubella is a togavirus spread through respiratory transmission. Viral reproduction occurs in the nasopharynx followed by a generalized viremia. The incubation period for rubella is 14 days followed by a prodromal phase lasting from 1 to 5 days. A maculopapular rash then occurs starting on the face, spreading to the entire body. This is often accompanied by arthralgias and arthritis. Rare complications include encephalitis and thrombocytopenic purpura. Perhaps the most devastating complication of rubella infection is congenital rubella syndrome. Rubella can cause a transplacental infection of the fetus resulting in spontaneous abortion, preterm delivery, deafness, cataracts, cardiac defects, microcephaly, mental retardation, and fetal death.

Epidemiology The primary goal of rubella vaccination is the prevention of congenital rubella syndrome.[46] Although endemic rubella spread has been eliminated since 2004, imported cases have been reported. Latino immigrants from regions without rubella vaccination programs have been the demographic group most often linked to rubella infection and congenital rubella syndrome in the United States over the past 20 years.[47]

Currently there are 2 live-attenuated forms of the vaccine available in the United States. There is the combined measles-mumps-rubella (MMR) vaccine and the same form combined with varicella (MMRV). Only MMR is used in adults. The ACIP recommends that the combined form (MMR) be used when any of the individual components is needed.

Immunogenicity and vaccine efficacy

The MMR vaccine has been proved effective at eliciting an appropriate antibody response and immunity for each of the vaccine components. Serologic and epidemiologic evidence indicates that vaccine-induced immunity after the MMR vaccines is long term and seems to be lifelong for most individuals. Measles antibodies develop in approximately 95% to 98% of individuals after 1 vaccination and in more than 99% of persons after 2 vaccinations. One dose of the MMR vaccine is 75% to 91% effective in producing protective antibody levels against mumps and greater than 95% effective in protecting against rubella. Seroconversion rates are similar whether the vaccine is given in single antigen form, as MMR, or MMRV.[48]

Vaccine highlights

Immunity to the MMR vaccine is long term and likely lifelong. Adults are presumed to be immune to MMR if they were born before 1957 (except health care workers), have had physician-diagnosed disease, have had appropriate immunization with live vaccine (an inactivated measles vaccine was available until 1967), or have laboratory evidence of immunity. Particular high-risk situations warrant the review of immune status in adults. Health care workers, students in postsecondary educational programs, and international travelers are at high risk of exposure to these diseases, and outbreaks have been associated with these conditions. Nonimmune individuals should receive at least 1 dose of live MMR vaccine. In high-risk situations (discussed previously), 2 doses should be administered. In addition, women of childbearing age should be assessed for rubella immunity. Nonimmune women should be immunized with MMR vaccine to avoid the risk of congenital rubella syndrome in their offspring.[41] Because MMR is a live vaccine, administration should occur 28 days before conception or on completion of pregnancy due to theoretic concerns for fetal rubella infection.[49]

SUMMARY

Immunizations remain one of the most effective clinical interventions available in modern medicine. Yet adult vaccination rates are significantly below acceptable levels, due to inadequacies in the health care system and challenges at the provider level. Primary care physicians face the responsibility of considering multiple aspects of an individual's health, environment, lifestyle, and occupation to immunize appropriately. This article outlines the appropriate use and indication of adult vaccines.

REFERENCES

1. Poland GA, Schaffner W. Immunization guidelines for adult patients: an annual update and a challenge. Ann Intern Med 2009;150(1):53–4.
2. Center for Disease Control, Prevention (CDC). Ten great public health achievements—United States, 1900-1999. MMWR Morb Mortal Wkly Rep 1999;48(12):241–3.
3. Maciosek MV, Coffield AB, Edwards NM, et al. Priorities among effective clinical preventive services: results of a systematic review and analysis. Am J Prev Med 2006;31:52–60.
4. Centers for Disease Control and Prevention. Coverage estimates for school entry vaccinations. Available at: http://www2.cdc.gov/nip/schoolsurv/nationalAvg5Year.asp. Accessed June 27, 2011.
5. Centers for Disease Control and Prevention. Influenza vaccination coverage levels. Available at: http://www.cdc.gov/flu/professionals/acip/coveragelevels.htm#tab3. Accessed June 27, 2011.
6. Centers for Disease Control and Prevention. TABLE: self-reported pneumococcal vaccination coverage trends 1989-2008 among adults, United States, National Health Interview Survey (NHIS). Available at: http://www.cdc.gov/flu/professionals/pdf/NHIS89_08ppvvaxtrendtab.pdf. Accessed June 27, 2011.
7. Hinman AR, Orenstein WA. Adult immunization: what can we learn from the childhood immunization program? Clin Infect Dis 2007;45:1532–5.
8. Hinman AR, Ross DA. Immunization registries can be building blocks for national health information systems. Health Aff (Milwood) 2010;29(4):676–82.
9. Task Force on Community Services. Recommendations regarding interventions to improve vaccination coverage in children, adolescents, and adults. Am J Prev Med 2000;18(Suppl 1):92–6.
10. Pickering LK, Baker CJ, Freed GL, et al. Immunization programs for infants, children, adolescents, and adults: clinical practice guidelines by the Infectious Diseases Society of America. Clin Infect Dis 2009;49:817–40.
11. Wendelboe A, Van Rie A, Salmaso S. Duration of immunity against pertussis after natural infection or vaccination. Pediatr Infect Dis J 2005;24:S58–61.
12. Centers for Disease Control, Prevention. Preventing tetanus, diphtheria, and pertussis among adults: use of tetanus toxoid, reduced diphtheria toxoid and acellular pertussis vaccine. Recommendations of the Advisory Committee on Immunization Practices (ACIP). MMWR Recomm Rep 2006;55(RR-17):1–33.
13. de Greeff SC, Mooi FR, Westerhof A, et al. Pertussis disease burden in the household: how to protect young infants. Clin Infect Dis 2010;50(10):1339–45.
14. AAFP. ACIP recommends tdap for pregnant women, removal of egg allergy as flu vaccine contraindication. Available at: http://www.aafp.org/online/en/

home/publications/news/news-now/health-of-the-public/20110629acipnewreqs.html. Accessed June 27, 2011.
15. Healthy People 2020, U.S. Department of Health and Human Services. Available at: http://www.healthypeople.gov/2020/default.aspx. Accessed June 27, 2011.
16. Nuorti JP, Butler JC, Farley MM, et al. Cigarette smoking and invasive pneumococcal disease. Active bacterial core surveillance team. N Engl J Med 2000;342(10):681–9.
17. Talbot TR, Hartert TV, Mitchel E, et al. Asthma as a risk factor for invasive pneumococcal disease. N Engl J Med 2005;352(20):2082–90.
18. Atkinson W, Wolfe S, Hamborsky J, et al, editors. Pneumococcal disease. epidemiology and prevention of vaccine-preventable diseases. Washington, DC: Public Health Foundation; 2009. p. 217–30.
19. Centers for Disease Control, Prevention. Updated recommendations for prevention of invasive pneumococcal disease among adults using the 23-valent pneumococcal polysaccharide vaccine (PPSV23). MMWR Morb Mortal Wkly Rep 2010;59:1102–6.
20. Atkinson W, Wolfe S, Hamborsky J, et al, editors. Meningococcal disease. Epidemiology and prevention of vaccine-preventable diseases. Washington, DC: Public Health Foundation; 2009. p. 177–88.
21. Centers for Disease Control, Prevention. Prevention and Control of Meningococcal Disease. Recommendations of the Advisory Committee on Immunization Practices (ACIP). MMWR Recomm Rep 2005;54(RR-7):1–21.
22. Weinstein LC, Buchanan EM, Hillson C, et al. Screening and prevention: cervical cancer. Prim Care 2009;36(3):559–74.
23. Parkin DM, Bray F. Chapter 2: the burden of HPV-related cancers. Vaccine 2006;24(Suppl 3):S11–25.
24. CDC. FDA Licensure of Quadrivalent Human Papillomavirus Vaccine (HPV4, Gardasil) for Use in Males and Guidance from the Advisory Committee on Immunization Practices (ACIP). Available at: http://www.cdc.gov/mmwr/preview/mmwrhtml/mm5920a5.htm?s_cid=mm5920a5_e. Accessed June 27, 2011.
25. Castellsagué X, Muñoz N, Pitisuttithum P, et al. End-of-study safety, immunogenicity, and efficacy of quadrivalent HPV (types 6, 11, 16, 18) recombinant vaccine in adult women 24–45 years of age. Advance online publication 31. Br J Cancer 2011;105(1):28–37.
26. Giuliano AR, Palefsky JM, Goldstone S, et al. Efficacy of quadrivalent HPV vaccine against HPV Infection and disease in males. N Engl J Med 2011;364(5):401–11.
27. Bleyer A. Cancer of the oral cavity and pharynx in young females: increasing incidence, role of human papilloma virus, and lack of survival improvement. Semin Oncol 2009;36(5):451–9.
28. Atkinson W, Wolfe S, Hamborsky J, et al, editors. Hepatitis A. Epidemiology and prevention of vaccine-preventable diseases. Washington, DC: Public Health Foundation; 2009. p. 85–96.
29. Klevens RM, Miller JT, Iqbal K, et al. The evolving epidemiology of hepatitis a in the United States: incidence and molecular epidemiology from population-based surveillance, 2005-2007. Arch Intern Med 2010;170(20):1811–8.
30. Center for Disease Control, Prevention. Prevention of Hepatitis A through active or passive immunization: recommendations of the Advisory Committee on Immunization Practices (ACIP). MMWR Recomm Rep 2006;55(RR-7):1–23.
31. Center for Disease Control, Prevention. A Comprehensive immunization strategy to eliminate transmission of Hepatitis B virus infection in the United States.

Recommendations of the Advisory Committee on Immunization Practices (ACIP). Part II: vaccination of adults. MMWR Recomm Rep 2006;55(RR16): 1–33.
32. Atkinson W, Wolfe S, Hamborsky J, et al, editors. Hepatitis B. Epidemiology and prevention of vaccine-preventable diseases. Washington, DC: Public Health Foundation; 2009. p. 99–122.
33. Center for Disease Control, Prevention. Prevention of varicella: recommendations of the Advisory Committee on Immunization Practices (ACIP). MMWR Recomm Rep 2007;56(No. RR-4):1–40.
34. Atkinson W, Wolfe S, Hamborsky J, et al, editors. Varicella. Epidemiology and prevention of vaccine-preventable diseases. Washington, DC: Public Health Foundation; 2009. p. 283–304.
35. Center for Disease Control, Prevention. Prevention of herpes zoster: recommendations of the Advisory Committee on Immunization Practices (ACIP). MMWR Recomm Rep 2008;57(RR-5):1–16.
36. Tseng H, Harpaz R, Bialek S. Herpes zoster vaccine in older adults and the risk of subsequent herpes zoster disease. JAMA 2011;305(2):160–6.
37. Atkinson W, Wolfe S, Hamborsky J, et al, editors. Influenza. Epidemiology and prevention of vaccine-preventable diseases. Washington, DC: Public Health Foundation; 2009. p. 135–56.
38. Centers for Disease Control, Prevention. Prevention and Control of Influenza with Vaccines. Recommendations of the Advisory Committee on Immunization Practices (ACIP). MMWR Recomm Rep 2010;59:1–62.
39. Zaman K, Roy E, Arifeen SE, et al. Effectiveness of maternal influenza immunization in mothers and infants. N Engl J Med 2008;359(15):1555–64.
40. Muszkat M, Greenbaum E, Ben-Yehuda A, et al. Local and systemic immune response in nursing-home elderly following intranasal or intramuscular immunization with inactivated influenza vaccine. Vaccine 2003;21(11–12):1180–6.
41. Centers for Disease Control, Prevention. In: Atkinson W, Wolfe S, Hamborsky J, editors. Measles. Epidemiology and prevention of vaccine-preventable diseases. 12th edition. Washington, DC: Public Health Foundation; 2011. p. 173–92.
42. Strebel PM, Papania MJ, Dayan GH, et al. Measles vaccine. In: Plotkin SA, Orenstein WA, Offit PA, editors. Vaccines. 5th edition. Philadelphia: Saunders Elsevier; 2008. p. 353–98.
43. Centers for Disease Control, Prevention. Update measles—United States, January—July 2008. MMWR Morb Mortal Wkly Rep 2008;57(33):893–6.
44. Plotkin SA, Rubin SA. Mumps vaccine. In: Plotkin SA, Orenstein WA, Offit PA, editors. Vaccines. 5th edition. Philadelphia: Saunders Elsevier; 2008. p. 435–65.
45. Centers for Disease Control, Prevention. In: Atkinson W, Wolfe S, Hamborsky J, editors. Mumps. Epidemiology and prevention of vaccine-preventable diseases. 12th edition. Washington, DC: Public Health Foundation; 2011. p. 205–14.
46. Rubella vaccines: WHO position paper. Weekly Epidemiological Record, 2011; 86(29):301–16. Available at: http://www.who.int/wer. Accessed August 28, 2011.
47. Centers for Disease Control, Prevention. In: Atkinson W, Wolfe S, Hamborsky J, editors. Rubella. Epidemiology and prevention of vaccine-preventable diseases. 12th edition. Washington, DC: Public Health Foundation; 2011. p. 275–90.
48. Vaccine preventable diseases. 12th edition. Available on-line at: http://www.cdc.gov/vaccines/pubs/pinkbook/pink-chapters.htm. Accessed June 27, 2011.
49. Centers for Disease Control. Notice to readers: revised ACIP recommendation for avoiding pregnancy after receiving a rubella-containing vaccine. MMWR Morb Mortal Wkly Rep 2001;50(49):1117.

Vaccine-Preventable Diseases and Foreign-Born Populations

Giang T. Nguyen, MD, MPH, MSCE[a,*], Marc Altshuler, MD[b]

KEYWORDS

• Immunization • Vaccine • Immigrant • Refugee
• Minority • Adoption

At the time of the 2000 census, foreign-born individuals accounted for 11.1% of the total US population.[1] By 2009, this percentage increased to 12%, totaling 36.7 million foreign-born individuals in the United States.[2] The US foreign-born population includes immigrants (legal permanent residents), humanitarian migrants (eg, refugees), temporary migrants (eg, students), and unauthorized migrants (undocumented individuals residing in the United States). Persons born abroad to American parents or born in Puerto Rico or other US Island Areas are not considered foreign born.[1]

Refugees constitute a special subset of the foreign-born population because of the sociopolitical factors leading to their migration. From 2000 to 2009, 618,090 refugees migrated to the United States from more than 60 different countries. The top 10 countries of origin were Cuba, the former Soviet Union, Somalia, former Yugoslavia, Burma, Iraq, Iran, Liberia, Sudan, and Vietnam. Refugees in the United States resettle in some regions more often than others, and the states with the largest number of resettled refugees are Florida, California, Texas, New York, and Minnesota.[3]

There is substantial evidence that many of the vaccine-preventable outbreaks in the United States have been directly related to disease importation. In 2008, close to 90% of the measles cases in the United States were either acquired overseas or imported cases, leading to 7 outbreaks and 135 infected persons.[4] Even though rubella disease is less severe than measles, congenital rubella syndrome can be devastating and life threatening. Fortunately, only 2 cases were reported in the United States in 2009.[5] However, in 1 of the 2 cases, the individual was traveling throughout her first trimester

Funding Support: None.
Financial Disclosures/Conflicts of Interest: the authors have nothing to disclose.
[a] Department of Family Medicine and Community Health, University of Pennsylvania, 3400 Spruce Street, 2 Gates/HUP, Philadelphia, PA 19104, USA
[b] Department of Family and Community Medicine, Thomas Jefferson University, 833 Chestnut Street, Suite 301, Philadelphia, PA 19107, USA
* Corresponding author.
E-mail address: nguyeng@uphs.upenn.edu

Prim Care Clin Office Pract 38 (2011) 633–642
doi:10.1016/j.pop.2011.07.004 primarycare.theclinics.com
0095-4543/11/$ – see front matter

in India and China. For these reasons, the Congress has mandated vaccinations for immigrant populations in the United States to decrease the public health burden from imported vaccine-preventable diseases.

As a whole, foreign-born individuals have unique immunization-related needs that can be influenced by country of origin, age of arrival to the United States, and circumstances surrounding their migration (eg, refugees/asylees, adoptees). Primary care physicians must be aware of these needs and must be comfortable providing the appropriate services to this population.

START WITH THE BASICS

In the primary care setting, foreign-born patients may present with complicated medical and social histories, and it is important to keep in mind the standard age-appropriate preventive care recommendations that apply to all patients. Compared with their US cohorts, foreign-born individuals may have more difficulty accessing health care because of cultural and linguistic barriers.[6,7] Foreign-born patients may be more likely to access health care for acute care rather than health maintenance, so sick visits should be viewed as an opportunity to provide these important services, including vaccination. Many of these patients do not return for a separate health maintenance visit, even if the recommendation is made. In many developing countries, the concept of a health maintenance visit is largely unknown, so the idea of returning to simply discuss wellness issues may be viewed with skepticism, even if patients outwardly voice agreement with the follow-up plan. Vaccination should not be delayed because of mild respiratory tract infections or other acute illness, although vaccination should be deferred for moderate or severe illness.[8]

ASSESSING RISK: IMPORTANT VACCINE-PREVENTABLE DISEASES FOR FOREIGN-BORN POPULATIONS

Knowing a patient's country of origin can help to assess the patient's level of risk for certain preventable diseases. Unfortunately, for the sake of examining the incidence of disease in these populations, immigrants are usually grouped together as a single unit, even though the incidence and prevalence of diseases differ among particular subgroups. In addition, it is also important for the primary care physician to have a general understanding of the cultural norms in these individuals to better assess an individual's risk for disease (ie, the risk of sexually transmitted infections in populations with a high prevalence of sexual abuse).

Despite near-total eradication of numerous vaccine-preventable diseases in the United States, the rest of the world has not been as fortunate. In 2002, the World Health Organization (WHO) estimated that 14% (1.4 million deaths) of the total global mortality in children younger than 5 years was because of disease that could have been prevented with routine vaccination. The distribution of these deaths is seen in **Fig. 1**.[9] In the following sections, the authors focus specifically on tuberculosis (TB), viral hepatitis, and human papillomavirus (HPV). These conditions were selected for special emphasis because of the greater burden of disease caused by these infections among immigrant populations.

INFECTIOUS DISEASE BURDEN

Tuberculosis

TB is very common in much of the world, with the continent of Africa having the largest number of high-prevalence nations. Continents with lowest rates of TB include North

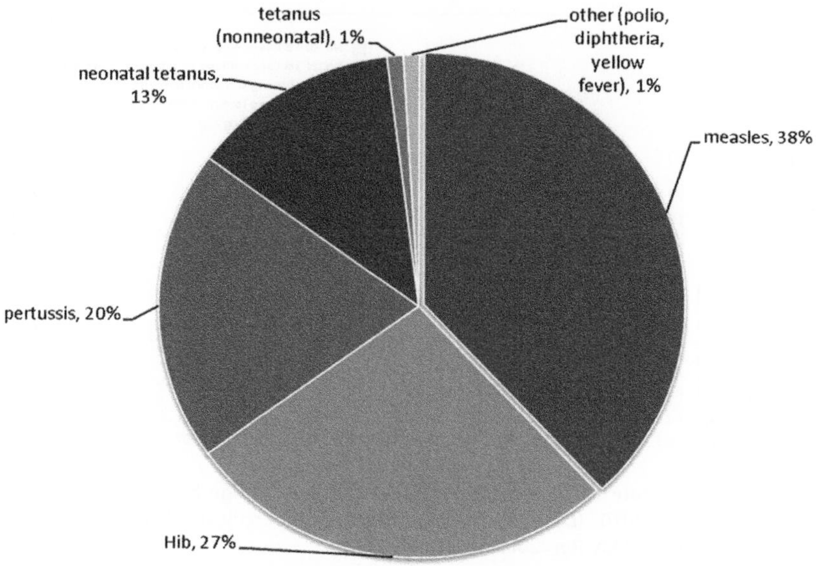

Fig. 1. Distribution of estimated annual deaths from vaccine-preventable diseases, 2002. (*Data from* World Health Organization. Vaccine preventable diseases. 2011 Internet Web page. Available at: http://www.who.int/immunization_monitoring/diseases/en/. Accessed June 20, 2011.)

America, Europe, and Australia. According to the WHO, the country with the highest incidence for the combined years of 2007 to 2008 was Swaziland in southern Africa, with an incidence of 510 per 100,000 population (compared with 2 per 100,000 in the United States).[10]

Although immunization against TB is not commonly performed (and not routinely recommended) in the United States,[11] there are many parts of the world where for years children have been routinely given the BCG vaccine to prevent TB. Although the vaccine has not been shown to make a large epidemiologic impact on TB infection per se, it seems to confer some protection against serious TB disease among children and may also protect against the development of leprosy.[12] Prior vaccination with BCG can sometimes result in false-positive results for the standard tuberculin skin test (TST).[13] Because many foreign-born individuals come from areas with endemic TB, further testing is necessary to identify these high-risk individuals.

Two newer blood tests serve as alternatives to the TST and are unaffected by prior BCG vaccination: the enzyme-linked immunosorbent assay–based QuantiFERON-TB Gold, which measures interferon-γ concentration in supernatant, and the enzyme-linked immunospot (ELISpot; T-SPOT TB), which enumerates interferon-γ–secreting T cells. Both tests have better specificity than the TST, although the immunospot test seems to have a higher sensitivity for detecting latent TB infection.[13] Despite decreases in active TB cases for US-born individuals, the numbers of active TB cases among foreign-born individuals in the United States are still relatively elevated and have remained stable over the years (**Figs. 2** and **3**). Identification and treatment of these individuals is necessary to decrease the burden of TB disease. Unfortunately, simple inexpensive point-of-care tests with this level of sensitivity and specificity are still not available.[14]

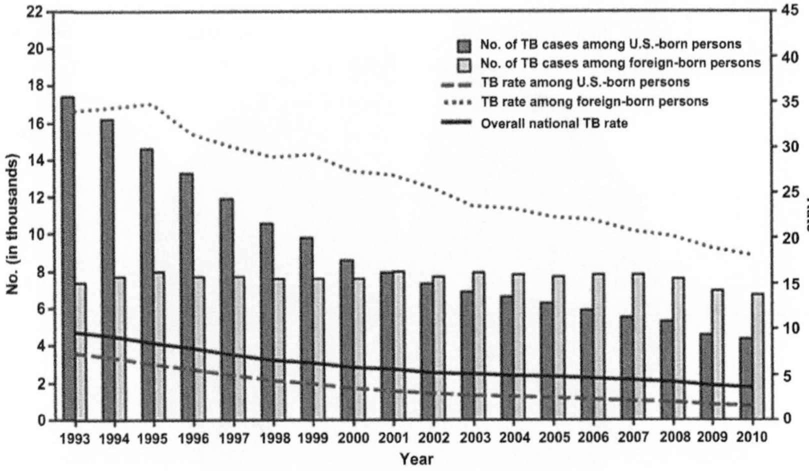

Fig. 2. Number and rate of TB cases among US-born and foreign-born persons by year—United States, 1993–2010. (*Data from* CDC. Trends in tuberculosis—United States, 2008. MMWR Morb Mortal Wkly Rep 2009;58(10);249–53.)

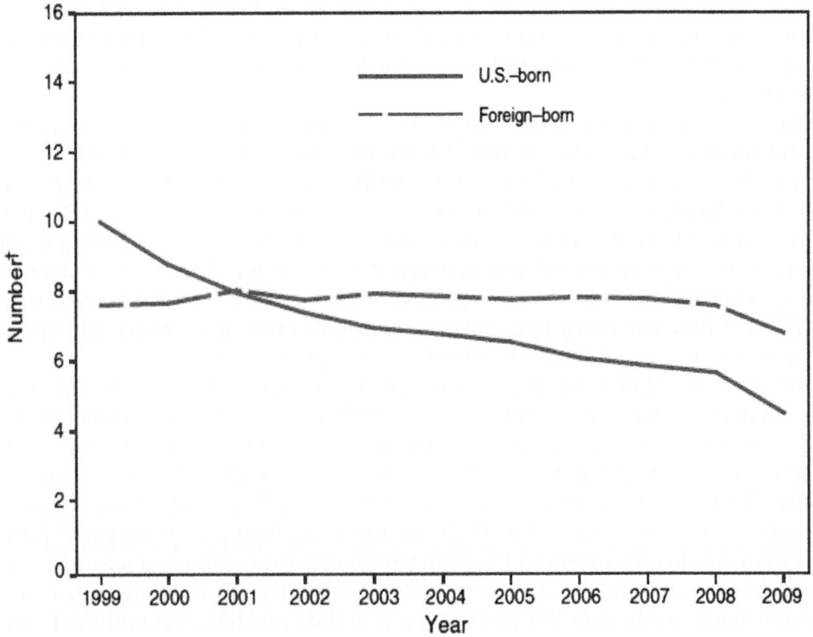

Fig. 3. Number of TB cases reported among US-born and foreign-born individuals (1999–2009). (*Data from* CDC. Summary of notifiable diseases—United States, 2009. MMWR Morb Mortal Wkly Rep 2011;58(53):1–100.)

Hepatitis A

Since the introduction of hepatitis A vaccination in 1995, cases of hepatitis A virus (HAV) in the United States have decreased 84%.[15] However, hepatitis A remains endemic in many parts of the world. High-prevalence regions include sub-Saharan Africa and parts of south Asia, where it is estimated that 90% or more of the population have serologic evidence of infection by age 10 years. Intermediate prevalence occurs in Latin America, northern Africa, and the Middle East (≥50% with evidence of infection by age 15 years).[16] Chronic hepatitis A has not been reported, although 10% to 20% of symptomatic patients experience a prolonged or relapsing course.[17] For all patients, but particularly those who have recently traveled from high-risk regions, hepatitis A should be considered in the setting of symptoms such as abdominal pain, fatigue, nausea, anorexia, urticaria, and jaundice. Infected children, however, may be asymptomatic; only about 30% of infected children exhibit symptoms (often non-specific flu-like symptoms), and viral shedding may continue in their stools for 6 months.[17]

Hepatitis B

Hepatitis B is endemic in many regions of the world as well, including much of Eastern Europe, Asia, Africa, the Middle East, and the Pacific Islands (**Fig. 4**). Chronic hepatitis B infection can result in liver failure, cirrhosis, and hepatocellular carcinoma. Only 0.3% to 0.5% of the US population is chronically infected with hepatitis B, but, among foreign-born individuals in the US, prevalence is 1.0% to 2.6%.[18]

People who come from countries with a hepatitis B prevalence of 2% or more are at greatest risk for both active and chronic hepatitis B infection. These individuals should be screened via hepatitis B surface antigen (HBsAg) testing and immunized if they are

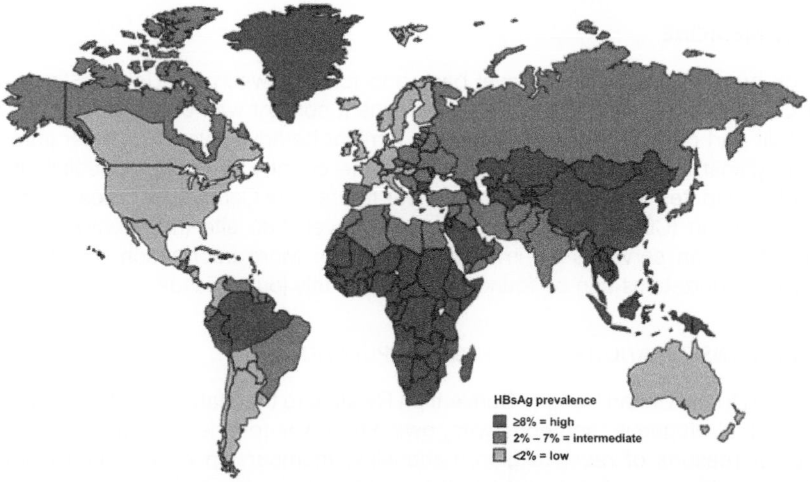

Fig. 4. Geographic distribution of chronic hepatitis B virus infection—worldwide, 2006. For multiple countries, estimates of prevalence of B surface antigen (HBsAg), a marker of chronic HBV infection, are based on limited data and might not reflect current prevalence in countries that have implemented childhood hepatitis B vaccination. In addition, HBsAg prevalence might vary within countries by subpopulation and locality. (*Data from* Weinbaum CM, Williams I, Mast EE, et al. Recommendations for identification and public health management of persons with chronic hepatitis B virus infection. MMWR Morb Mortal Wkly Rep 2008;57(RR08):1–20.)

not infected (unless there is documentation that there has been prior completion of the immunization series). For foreign-born persons from high-risk countries, HBsAg testing is warranted even when there is a documented history of immunization because it is possible that infection could have occurred before immunization. In addition, testing is also recommended for US-born persons who were not vaccinated as infants and whose parents were born in regions with a hepatitis B virus (HBV) endemicity of 8% or more (eg, Peru, northern Brazil, Greenland, sub-Saharan Africa, Saudi Arabia, and much of Asia and the Pacific Islands).[18] For individuals with unknown hepatitis B immunization history, it is reasonable to consider testing for hepatitis B surface antibody before deciding to immunize; however, if the cost of serologic testing exceeds the cost of immunization, it might be more cost effective merely to vaccinate.

Human Papillomavirus

There is clear evidence in the medical literature to support the direct relationship that human papillomavirus (HPV) has on the development of cancer, including cervical, vulvar, anal, penile, and oropharyngeal cancers. HPV has been recognized as the cause of essentially all cervical cancers.[19–21] Even though the number of cervical cancer cases in the United States is very low, cervical cancer affects many women worldwide.[22,23] HPV vaccines that are available in the United States and other countries have been shown to prevent the transmission of the high-risk HPV subtypes that pose the greatest risk to the development of cervical cancer.[23] Many foreign-born individuals are likely to be behind in cervical cancer screening. Administration of the HPV vaccine to this population at the earliest visit to the health care provider is essential in lowering the incidence of cervical cancer. However, the HPV immunization does not prevent infection of all oncogenic HPV subtypes (only 16 and 18) nor does it treat infections that have already occurred before immunization. Therefore, Papanicolaou testing is still an essential component in the prevention of cervical cancer, regardless of HPV immunization status.

TRAVEL MEDICINE

Foreign-born individuals may travel back and forth between the United States and their country of origin, or they may have frequent contact with other people who are from that part of the world. Consequently, it might be advisable to consider immunization against illnesses that are common in the country of origin, especially if the patient anticipates traveling there in the near future. The Centers for Disease Control and Prevention (CDC) has a comprehensive travel Web site (http://www.cdc.gov/travel/) that can serve as an important resource. More information about travel-related immunizations can be found elsewhere in this journal issue.

SPECIAL CONSIDERATIONS FOR REFUGEE POPULATIONS

According to the United Nations Convention Relating to the Status of Refugees (Article 1A: 1951), a refugee is "someone who, owing to a well-founded fear of being persecuted for reasons of race, religion, nationality, membership of a particular social group, or political opinion, is outside the country of his nationality, and is unable to or, owing to such fear, is unwilling to avail himself of the protection of that country."[24]

Approximately 80,000 refugees arrive annually into the United States, with more than 2 million arrivals since 1980.[25] Refugees bring a unique set of medical issues and conditions that must be addressed by the treating health care provider. Before arrival in the United States, all refugees undergo an overseas medical examination with the purpose of identifying any diseases (ie, active TB, leprosy) that would preclude travel to the United States. Depending on the country of origin, vaccinations may also be provided at the time of this examination.

According to the Immigration and Nationality Act (Section 212), any individual seeking admission to the United States, either as an incoming immigrant or as an immigrant seeking an adjustment of status for permanent US residence (green card), is ineligible for admission to the United States if they are unable to present the appropriate documentation of having received vaccinations against "vaccine-preventable diseases, which shall include at least the following diseases: Mumps, measles, rubella, polio, tetanus and diphtheria toxoids, pertussis, *Haemophilus influenzae* type B, and hepatitis B, and any other vaccinations against vaccine-preventable diseases recommended by the Advisory Committee on Immunization Practices (ACIP)." Vaccinations given overseas are considered acceptable if they have been given at the appropriate intervals and age guidelines.

All refugees are eligible for adjustment of status after they have lived in the United States for 1 year. For this reason, vaccination is an essential piece in the medical care of newly arrived refugees to the United States. In addition, for refugee children to attend school in the United States, they must have either appropriate documentation of vaccinations provided overseas or initiated the vaccination series in the United States. Because of the large number of vaccinations that are required for both children and adults, health care providers need to be very familiar with the CDC's guidelines on vaccinations, including child, adolescent, adult, and catch-up schedules. As of December 14, 2009, the CDC has new criteria that will be used to decide which vaccines will be required as part of the immigration process. The criteria are as follows:

1. The vaccine must be an age-appropriate vaccine as recommended by the Advisory Committee on Immunization Practices for the general US population.
2. At least 1 of the following:
   - The vaccine must protect against a disease that has the potential to cause an outbreak.
   - The vaccine must protect against a disease that has been eliminated in the United States or is in the process for elimination in the United States.

Any changes made by the CDC will be reflected in the CDC's Technical Instructions for Panel Physicians for Vaccinations (http://www.cdc.gov/immigrantrefugeehealth). The current requirements for routine vaccination during the immigration process are given in **Table 1**.

INTERNATIONAL ADOPTEES AND OTHERS RECEIVING VACCINATION OUTSIDE THE UNITED STATES

Evidence of immunization before coming to the United States must be proved by written documentation, with the exception of influenza and pneumococcal polysaccharide vaccine, for which verbal history is acceptable. Adequate protection is most likely if the vaccination history closely matches the US immunization schedule regarding age of administration and immunization interval. Even with documented immunizations, however, it is possible that serologic testing may reveal inadequate protection. Repeating of immunizations according to the catch-up schedule is an appropriate option to ensure protection.[8]

Vaccination/revaccination is recommended for measles, mumps, and rubella (MMR) and polio. In addition, age-appropriate vaccination/revaccination is recommended for *Haemophilus influenzae* type b, HAV, HBV (along with HBsAg testing), varicella (if lacking evidence of immunity), pneumococcal conjugate, rotavirus, HPV, and zoster infection. Alternatively, MMR, poliovirus, and HAV immunity can be determined through serologic testing before deciding to administer these vaccines.[8]

Table 1
Requirements for routine vaccination of immigrants examined overseas who are not fully vaccinated or lack documentation

	Age						
Vaccine	**Birth–1 Month**	**2–11 Months**	**12 Months–6 Years**	**7–10 Years**	**11–17 Years**	**18–64 Years**	**≥65 Years**
DTP/DTaP/DT	NO	YES		NO			
Td/Tdap	NO			YES if 7 years and older (for Td); if 10 years through 64 years (for Tdap- see ACIP schedule); if 65 years and older (for Td)			
Polio (IPV/OPV)	NO	YES				NO	
Measles, Mumps, and Rubella	NO		yes, if born in 1957 or later			NO, if born before 1957	
Rotavirus	NO	YES, if 6 weeks to 8 months	NO				
Hib	NO	YES, if 2 months through 59 months		NO			
Hepatitis A	NO		YES, if 12 months through 23 months	NO			
Hepatitis B	YES, birth through 18 years					NO	
Meningococcal (MCV4)	NO				YES, if 11 years through 18 years	NO	
Varicella	NO		YES				
Pneumococcal	NO	YES, if 2 months through 59 months (for PCV)		NO			YES (for PPV)
influenza	NO	YES, 6 months and older (annually each flu season)					

Abbreviations: DT, pediatric formulation diphtheria and tetanus toxoids; DTaP, diphtheria and tetanus toxoids and acellular pertussis vaccine; DTP, diphtheria and tetanus toxoids and pertussis vaccine; Hib, Haemophilus influenzae type b conjugate vaccine; IPV, inactivated poliovirus vaccine (killed); MCV, meningococcal conjugate vaccine; OPV, orai poliovirus vaccine (live); PCV, pneumococcal conjugate vaccine; PPV, pneumococcal polysaccharide vaccine; Tdap, adolescent and adult formulation tetanus and diphtheria toxoids and acellular pertussis vaccine (Boostrix for persons aged 10 to 64 years; Adacel for persons aged 11 to 64 years); Td, adult formulation tetanus and diphtheria toxoids.

Adapted from ACIP recommendations; and *Data from* CDC. 2009 technical instructions for panel physicians for vaccinations. 2010. Internet Web page. Available at: http://www.cdc.gov/immigrantrefugeehealth/exams/ti/panel/vaccination-panel-technical-instructions.html. Accessed June 24, 2011.

Revaccination is also recommended for diphtheria and tetanus toxoids and acellular pertussis vaccine (DTaP), but adverse local reactions are more common after the fourth or fifth dose. Therefore, if a severe local reaction occurs, IgG titers for tetanus and diphtheria toxins should be obtained before deciding to proceed with additional DTaP administrations (although serologic tests exist for tetanus/diphtheria, there are no currently available serologic tests to confirm adequate immunity against pertussis). For foreign-born children with 3 or more documented doses of DTaP before coming to the United States, it is also appropriate to do tetanus/diphtheria serologic testing at initial presentation or 1 month after a booster dose. If adequate immunity is demonstrated, only standard age-appropriate immunizations are necessary after that point. For older persons, adolescent and adult formulation tetanus and diphtheria toxoids and acellular pertussis vaccine should be administered as appropriate based on standard guidelines.[8]

SUMMARY

Despite the great progress that has been made in the United States in the last century with vaccine-preventable diseases, significant morbidity and mortality is seen throughout the world in individuals who have not been vaccinated. As the foreign-born population in the United States continues to increase, primary care physicians must feel comfortable treating these individuals in a culturally and linguistically appropriate manner.

REFERENCES

1. USA quickfacts from the US Census Bureau. Internet Web page. Last updated November 4, 2010. Available at: http://quickfacts.census.gov/qfd/states/00000.html. US Census Bureau; 2010. Accessed March 17, 2011.
2. Foreign-born population of the United States current population survey—March 2009. US Census Bureau; 2010. Available at: http://www.census.gov/population/www/socdemo/foreign/cps2009.html#cit. Accessed April 28, 2011.
3. Eckstein B. Primary care for refugees. Am Fam Physician 2011;83(4):429–36.
4. Grigg M, Brzezny A, Dawson J, et al. Update: measles—United States, January–July 2008. MMWR Morb Mortal Wkly Rep 2008;57(33):893–6.
5. CDC. Summary of notifiable diseases—United States, 2009. MMWR Morb Mortal Wkly Rep 2011;58(53):1–100.
6. Mohanty S, Woolhandler S, Himmelstein DU, et al. Healthcare expenditures of immigrants in the United States: a nationally representative analysis. Am J Public Health 2005;95(8):1431–8.
7. Kandula NR, Kersey M, Lurie N. Assuring the health of immigrants: what the leading health indicators tell us. Annu Rev Public Health 2004;25:357–76.
8. CDC. General recommendations on immunization: recommendations of the Advisory Committee on Immunization Practices (ACIP). MMWR Recomm Rep 2011;60(RR2):1–64.
9. Vaccine preventable diseases. Internet Web page. Available at: http://www.who.int/immunization_monitoring/diseases/en/. World Health Organization; 2011. Accessed June 20, 2011.
10. International tuberculosis incidence rates. Internet Web page. Available at: http://www.phac-aspc.gc.ca/tbpc-latb/itir-eng.php. World Health Organization; 2010. Accessed March 17, 2011.
11. CDC. The role of BCG vaccine in the prevention and control of tuberculosis in the United States: a joint statement by the Advisory Council for the Elimination of

Tuberculosis and the Advisory Committee on Immunization Practices. MMWR Recomm Rep 1996;45(RR-4):1–18.
12. CDC. Development of new vaccines for tuberculosis: recommendations of the Advisory Council for the Elimination of Tuberculosis (ACET). MMWR Recomm Rep 1998;47(RR13):1–6.
13. Lalvani A. Diagnosing tuberculosis infection in the 21st century: new tools to tackle an old enemy. Chest 2007;131(6):1898–906.
14. Wallis RS, Pai M, Menzies D, et al. Biomarkers and diagnostics for tuberculosis: progress, needs, and translation into practice. Lancet 2010;375(9729):1920–37.
15. CDC. Hepatitis awareness month—special issue. MMWR Morb Mortal Wkly Rep 2006;55(18):505–28.
16. Jacobsen KH, Wiersma ST. Hepatitis A virus seroprevalence by age and world region, 1990 and 2005. Vaccine 2010;28(41):6653–7.
17. Brundage SC, Fitzpatrick AN. Hepatitis A. Am Fam Physician 2006;73(12): 2162–8.
18. Weinbaum CM, Williams I, Mast EE, et al. Recommendations for identification and public health management of persons with chronic hepatitis B virus infection. MMWR Morb Mortal Wkly Rep 2008;57(RR08):1–20.
19. Parkin DM. The global health burden of infection-associated cancers in the year 2002. Int J Cancer 2006;118(12):3030–44.
20. U.S. Cancer Statistics Working Group. United States cancer statistics: 1999–2007 incidence and mortality. Atlanta (GA): Department of Health and Human Services, Centers for Disease Control and Prevention, and National Cancer Institute; 2010.
21. D'Souza G, Kreimer AR, Viscidi R, et al. Case-control study of human papillomavirus and oropharyngeal cancer. N Engl J Med 2007;356(19):1944–56.
22. WHO. Human papillomavirus and related cancers. Barcelona (Spain): World Health Organization; 2010.
23. Garland SM, Hernandez-Avila M, Wheeler CM, et al. Quadrivalent vaccine against human papillomavirus to prevent anogenital diseases. N Engl J Med 2007;356(19):1928–43.
24. Internet Web page. United Nations for High Commissioner for Refugees (UNHCR); 2010. Available at:. http://www.unhcr.org/3b66c2aa10.html. Accessed June 19, 2011.
25. Anonymous. Report to Congress: proposed refugee admission for fiscal year 2011. Washington, DC: U.S. Department of State, U.S. Department of Homeland Security, U.S. Department of Health and Human Services; 2010.

Immunization in Travel Medicine

Suzanne Moore Shepherd, MD, MS, DTM&H*,
William Hudson Shoff, MD, DTM&H

KEYWORDS

• Travel medicine • Pretravel consultation • Immunization
• Tropical medicine

Health issues related to travel, conquest, and immigration are not new.[1–3] Imported plagues, including the Black Death, decimated Europe during the Middle Ages, with the resultant practice of quarantine developed in Italy and widely practiced in the ports of fourteenth-century Europe. Smallpox, measles, and other diseases introduced by Europeans ravaged native populations in the Americas. Infections, such as plague and smallpox, have been purposefully introduced to aid conquest of native peoples and subdue enemy combatants. In the last 2 centuries, returning ill travelers, military personnel, and expatriates received treatment in medical facilities specializing in tropical diseases and provided significant impetus to vaccine development.

We live in an increasingly populous and mobile world than experienced by past generations. In the last 2 centuries, the global population has grown from less than 1 billion to more than 6 billion. Population mobility has increased 100-fold since 1960. Travelers can now return to their home country from the most remote locations within 2 days. In 2005, the World Tourism Organization reported 783 million international arrivals per year, with just less than half involving countries outside of Europe. Yearly, 80 million people travel from relatively sanitary, temperate, industrialized nations to the tropical and developing world, increasingly to more remote locations. Travel, increasingly felt to be part of an educated and desirable lifestyle, is available to a wider segment of the population by air and cruise ships. International travel has not shown a significant decline despite economic downturns, increasing fares, and worldwide unrest. The latest available data from 2006 denote Europe to be the leader in annual trip volume, with a total of 475 million travelers internationally, most commonly within Europe (402.1 million), and to a lesser extent to the Americas (24 million), Asia and the Pacific (21.2 million), Africa (16.8 million), and the Middle East (11.2 million) (UN World Tourism Organization: http://www.unwto.org).

Neither author has any financial interests or conflicts of interest to disclose.
Department of Emergency Medicine, PENN Travel Medicine, Hospital of the University of Pennsylvania, 3400 Spruce Street, Philadelphia, PA 19104, USA
* Corresponding author.
E-mail address: suzanne.shepherd@uphs.upenn.edu

Prim Care Clin Office Pract 38 (2011) 643–679
doi:10.1016/j.pop.2011.07.005 **primarycare.theclinics.com**

Travelers are frequently unaware of health and safety risks posed by travel and the availability of pretravel consultation.[4,5] Travel-related risks are usually not discussed by travel agents. Immigrant populations increasingly return to their birth countries to visit friends and relatives (VFRs) often not seeking pretravel consultation because of mistaken belief in their continuing immunity to endemic infections.[6]

Reported morbidity among travelers varies considerably; however, some health impairment is reported by up to 75% of short-term travelers to developing countries, with traveler's diarrhea the most common complaint.[7] On a typical 2-week trip, travelers miss an average of 3 days of planned activities because of illness. Approximately 1 in 5 travelers visits a physician on return.[5] Travelers, immigrants, and refugees can rapidly and unexpectedly introduce new and reemerging infections to those who they interact with during return travel and into their home communities. Over the last decade, because of the growth of tourism, humanitarian aid, religious pilgrimages, military deployment, educational and business travel, and immigration and refugee placement, the global health community has increasingly faced the challenges brought on by the emergence and rapid worldwide spread of novel viruses, such as severe acute respiratory syndrome; novel influenza strains, such as H1N1; and other bacterial and parasitic microorganisms, such as *Plasmodium knowlesi* malaria and increasing drug resistance in organisms such as *P falciparum*, *Neisseria gonorrheae*, and *Mycobacterium tuberculosis*.

Only 1% to 3.6% of deaths in travelers are because of infectious diseases; however, the risk of acute and chronic health issues in individual travelers and the risk of global pathogen spread mandate health care provider attention to the prevention, recognition, treatment, and control of these illnesses. Malaria, the most common infectious cause of death among travelers, is easily prevented with appropriate awareness and precautions. Increasingly, issues of special needs must be addressed to travelers, including pregnancy, human immunodeficiency virus, organ transplantation, and physical disabilities. Travel health care providers need to be knowledgeable and experienced when counseling patients regarding relative risk and preventative measures for the wide variety of health and safety issues that they will face during their travel, to ask an appropriate travel and immigration history, and to diagnose and treat illnesses presenting in travelers, immigrants, and refugees.[8,9]

In response to these specialized concerns, a new multidisciplinary medical specialty, travel medicine, emerged in 1988. In 1991, the International Society of Travel Medicine (ISTM; http://www.istm.org) was formed during the Second International Conference in Atlanta, Georgia. In 2010, the 11th International Conference, held in Budapest, Hungary, attracted more than 2000 participants from 65 countries. Travel medicine initially focused on tropical medicine concerns; however, it now encompasses the gamut of travel-related issues, including epidemiology and preventative medicine, wilderness and environmental medical issues, occupational medicine concerns, migrant medicine, medical tourism, international health, and personal safety, as well as the protection of local and global communities in which individuals live, work, and travel. More recently, robust systematically collected data collaboratively obtained by specialized travel/tropical medicine networks, such as TropNet Europe (http://www.tropnet.net), EuroTravNet (http://www.eurotravnet.eu), and GeoSentinel (http://www.geosentinel.org), in conjunction with the European Center for Disease Prevention and Control and the US Centers for Disease Control and Prevention (CDC), have been found to be effective sentinels for early detection and trending of travel-related diseases.[7–9]

Travel medicine providers include tropical medicine specialists, specialized travel medicine services, adult and pediatric general practice providers, occupational medicine practitioners, and pharmacists. In the United States, surveys indicate that 38% of practitioners train in family or general internal medicine, whereas in Canada, approximately 54% of practitioners train in family medicine.[10] Travel and tropical medicine training has been increasingly embraced in emergency medicine over the last 20 years because of the escalating numbers of immigrants, refugees, and travelers presenting to emergency departments for care.[11] At present, few guidelines regarding certification and qualifications required to practice travel medicine exist. The Glasgow Diploma in Travel Medicine was the first diplomate course (DTM&H) offered by the Communicable Diseases Unit of the University of Glasgow in 1996. Several recognized courses are currently offered worldwide. Since 2003, ISTM has offered a voluntary Certificate of Knowledge Examination, which requires training and/or practice prerequisites. In 2010, the Royal College of Physicians and Surgeons of Glasgow introduced a formal 2-part examination to assess the knowledge of trained and experienced practitioners. Licensure to provide yellow fever vaccine is largely regulated by national or regional health care authorities in Europe and the United States. The CDC publishes the *Health Information for International Travel* (the Yellow Book), which serves as a reference, including updated malaria prophylaxis and treatment guidelines, for those advising international travelers about health risks (http://wwwnc.cdc.gov/travel/content/yellowbook/home-2010.aspx). Similar guidelines are available from several other national health services and specialty societies, such as the Public Health Agency of Canada's Travel Health Guidelines (http://www.phac-aspc.gc.ca/tmp-pmv/) and Health Protection Scotland's Travax Web site (http://www.travax.nhs.uk). Rigorous structured continuing medical education, including outpatient clinic and hospital rounds, didactic lectures, and laboratory work, is provided in many tropical countries worldwide by specialty organizations and tropical medicine consultants. Multiple studies underline the importance of appropriate training, experience, and ongoing education in providing individuals with proper peritravel care.[12–14]

TRAVEL MEDICINE PRACTICE

In general, travel medicine practice involves education and care of the traveler, before, during, and after a trip or more-prolonged stay in another country, to maintain traveler's well-being and safety and avoid importation of infectious agents. As noted, disease surveillance and care of migrants and refugees are becoming increasingly important additions to this practice. The pretravel consultation begins with an evaluation of the health and immunization status of the traveler and concludes with an assessment and a plan based on the itinerary-based risk. A growing number of decision-support resources and tools are available to facilitate this process, including government travel advice sites, Travax, Tropimed, and Gideon. Prevention of individual diseases is addressed by a combination of patient education, vaccination, provision of chemoprophylaxis, use of methods to avoid insect exposure, food and water precautions, provision of medication for self-treatment of certain illnesses, and provision of travel and evacuation insurance if desired. Individual recommendations are based on epidemiologically determined likelihood of injury and disease occurrence in an individual area and the individual traveler's health, experience, health belief model, and tolerance of risk.[15] At times, pretravel consultation may provide a cogent argument for travel postponement, as with pregnant women planning travel to malarial areas.

PRETRAVEL CONSULTATION

Routine medical and dental care should be updated before a trip. Patients are advised to carry a sufficient supply of required medications with them, because those drugs purchased overseas may not be the same drug, may not be manufactured to similar standards as those available in developed countries, or may contain counterfeit medications or contaminants. Detailed planning, equipment, and medications for large and specialized groups and expeditions are beyond the scope of this article but are readily available from several articles, texts, and on-line information sites provided by both the ISTM and the Wilderness Medicine Society.

Ideally, the initial pretravel consultation should occur at least 4 to 6 weeks before the patient's departure to allow adequate time for serial immunizations and immunizations to take effect, to begin antimalarials that must be started before arrival in endemic areas, and for assessment of potential adverse reactions to vaccinations and medications. If a traveler has less time before travel, it remains important to see a provider for necessary vaccines, antimalarials, other medications, and counseling. Some medications may cause vaccine interactions or interfere with vaccine-derived immune protection. For example, an interval of at least 10 days should be scheduled between a dose of oral cholera vaccine and the initial dose of chloroquine or mefloquine. In general, attenuated live virus vaccines and bacterial vaccines are contraindicated in persons with altered immune competence and during pregnancy.[16–18] Multiple vaccines may be given at different sites during the same visit, limited by the traveler's anticipated tolerance for multiple injections and minor side effects. Up to 6 live virus vaccines may be given on the same day without interfering with immune efficacy; otherwise live virus vaccine doses should be separated by at least 1 month. Some immunizations, such as hepatitis A, may be provided in an accelerated schedule.

Pretravel History

The individual's medical history, current medications and allergies, and immunizations are reviewed because these influence vaccine indications and potential contraindications.[18] For example, individuals with egg allergies have a potential contraindication to the vaccination for measles, mumps, rubella, yellow fever, influenza, and rabies. The pretravel history includes exploration and documentation of the individual's purposes for travel, specific travel itinerary, and duration, including discussion of planned or possible stopovers and side trips, with attention to seasonal and locale-specific variances in risk of infection and injury. For example, an individual traveling on business to Rio de Janeiro might wish to take a side trip to the Amazon, which will require additional counseling, vaccinations, and prophylaxis. The types of accommodation and likely styles of eating and drinking during the trip should be discussed relative to risk. Planned activities should also be reviewed relative to risk, for example, spelunking, white water rafting, fresh water and salt water swimming and diving, trekking in remote areas, and potential domestic and wild animal exposure. What degree of interaction will the traveler have with local populations? Will the traveler be engaged in agriculture, wildlife biology, construction, or local medical or humanitarian work? Will the individual travel to an area of unrest or conflict? Current outbreaks of disease and areas of violence and conflict, described on State Department, World Health Organization (WHO), CDC, Pan American Health Organization, and ProMed sites, also play important roles in pretravel counseling.

Immunizations

Immunization is the most common reason that patients seek pretravel consultations. Travelers to tropical and developing countries from Western Europe and North America are exposed to communicable diseases infrequently seen in their home countries because of generally high sanitation standards and mandatory childhood immunization. Appropriate immunization has been shown to increase the likelihood of a traveler remaining healthy. The CDC currently divides travel immunizations into 3 categories: routine, recommended, and required. First-time travelers may be dismayed at the number of vaccines recommended, the route of administration, and the cost. Because many vaccines are not covered by regular health insurance, vaccines and the relative risk of travel-related illness are prioritized for the traveler. Travelers may elect to obtain routine vaccinations from their primary care provider to maximize insurance coverage. All immunizations administered to travelers are recorded in a copy of the yellow booklet, *International Certificates of Vaccination*, recognized by the WHO, which should be kept with the individual's passport. A specific page validates yellow fever vaccination.

Routine immunizations before travel

Routine immunizations, such as those for tetanus, diphtheria, pertussis, measles, mumps, rubella, varicella, pneumococcus, and influenza, should be reviewed and updated as warranted. Travelers are counseled about the potential differences in influenza risk and likelihood of vaccine efficacy when traveling in semitropical and tropical areas than in temperate areas and between the northern and southern hemispheres. Because of the infrequent but continued presence of wild poliovirus and clinical polio in developing countries, the CDC currently recommends that adult travelers who have received a primary polio vaccination series with either inactivated poliovirus vaccine (IPV) or oral polio vaccine (OPV) should receive a single lifetime additional dose of IPV.[19] The CDC currently recommends that all adults (younger than 65 years) should receive 1 dose of Tdap (tetanus-diptheria-pertussis vaccine) as one of their recommended 10-year boosters, which is particularly relevant to the traveler because of the increased likelihood of exposure to diphtheria and pertussis in developing countries. Individuals born before 1958 are generally considered immune to measles and mumps. All individuals born after 1957 should have documentation of 1 or more doses of measles-mumps-rubella (MMR) vaccine unless they have medical contraindication, laboratory evidence of immunity to each of the 3 diseases, or documentation of provider-diagnosed measles or mumps. Individuals who received inactivated (killed) measles vaccine or measles vaccine of unknown type during the period from 1963 to 1967 should be revaccinated with 2 doses of measles vaccine. Because of a significant risk of measles exposure, a second MMR vaccine, administered a minimum of 28 days after the first, is recommended for adults who work in outbreak settings or in health care settings in developing countries or plan to travel internationally.[20]

Recommended vaccines before travel

Recommended vaccines include those that help to protect travelers from contracting illnesses present in other parts of the world and to prevent the importation of infectious diseases across international borders. Which vaccinations an individual will need depends on several factors, including the traveler's age and health status, previous immunization, the destination, the season of the year the individual will be traveling, the length of time an individual will spend in a specific area, whether a traveler will be spending time in rural areas, what activities the individual will engage in,[21–23] and whether the destination is currently experiencing disease outbreaks. For example, rabies preexposure prophylaxis is recommended for those travelers who will spend a significant time outdoors, especially in rural areas, or who anticipate activities such as spelunking, cycling, camping, or hiking. Rabies vaccination is also recommended for travelers with significant occupational risk (such as veterinarians); for long-term travelers and expatriates living in areas of significant exposure risk; and for travelers involved in any activities that might bring them into direct contact with bats, carnivores, and other mammals. Children are considered at higher risk for rabies exposure because they tend to interact with animals, may receive more bites, and may not report bites or exposures. See **Table 1** for a list of recommended vaccinations for travel to certain countries.

Table 1
Travel vaccines

Vaccine	Type	Administration	Booster Interval	Indications	Efficacy	Contraindications	Precautions	Comments	Side Effects
Cholera (OCV)-CVD 103-HgR (Orochol-E; Berna Biotech, Bern, Switzerland)	Live attenuated, derived from reference strain 569B (classical, O1, Inaba)	Oral, 1 dose	6-mo intervals for continued risk	No WHO regulation. 2 available that are considered safe and efficacious. Consider for long-term travel to endemic areas or to areas with active outbreaks	60%–90% in clinical studies	Not recommended for children younger than 2 y. Not recommended in pregnancy. Not recommended in immune deficiency and immuno-suppressive or antimitotic drugs	Travelers should still follow food and water precautions. Travelers with underlying gastric hypochlorhydria or partial resection or who take medications that block gastric acid production may have increased susceptibility to cholera.	Earliest onset of protective immunity 8 d after immunization Does not protect against *V cholerae* O139	Rare gastrointestinal
WC/rBS (Dukoral; SBL Powderject, Stockholm, Sweden)	Killed whole unit B subunit	Oral, 2 doses 10–14 d apart	6-mo intervals for continued risk	No WHO regulation. 2 available that are considered safe and efficacious	50%–86%	Not recommended for children younger than 2 y	Travelers should still follow food and water precautions. Travelers with underlying gastric hypochlorhydria or partial resection or who take medications that block gastric acid production may have increased susceptibility to cholera.	Earliest onset of protective immunity 10 d after the second dose Not available in United States. Available in Canada, Western Europe, South America, and Asia. Offers some protection against traveler's diarrhea because of cross-reactivity with heat-labile toxin. Does not protect against *V cholerae* O139 A variant WC/rBS is licensed in	Rare gastrointestinal

								Vietnam which contains no recombinant B-subunit, also administered in 2 doses, 1 wk apart	
Hepatitis A (HAV) (Havrix; GlaxoSmith-Kline Biologicals, Pittsburgh, PA, USA)	Inactivated HAV, derived from HM-175 viral strain	Intramuscular (IM) deltoid, 2 doses	0 and 6–12 mo (delay in booster dose up to 66 mo in testing did not seem to influence anamnestic immune response to the booster dose	Hepatitis A is a serious viral infection with fecal oral transmission, which is the leading cause of vaccine-preventable illness occurring among nonimmune international travelers. The incidence rate can be as high as 20 cases/1000 travelers/mo during adventure or rural travel, and 3–6 cases/1000 travelers/mo in those going to tourist areas and resorts, in developing countries.	90%–100% seropositivity rate	Not recommended for children younger than 1 y. Sensitivity to aluminum, aluminum hydroxy, or 2-phenoxy-ethanol		Available worldwide Protective immunity 2–4 wk following receipt 1st dose. 2nd dose confers lasting immunity >10y. Now included among routine immunizations in US for children Updated recommen-dations no longer call for dose IG when hepatitis A is given <2 wk before departure	Severe allergic reaction (eg, anaphylaxis) after a previous dose of any hepatitis A–containing vaccine, or to any component of HAVRIX, including neomycin. The most common adverse events are injection-site soreness (56% adults, 21% children) and headache (14% adults, <9% children)
HAV (VAQTA; Merck & Co, Inc, Whitehouse	Inactivated HAV, derived from CR-326F strain	IM deltoid, 2 doses	0 and 6–12 mo (delay in booster dose up to 66 mo in testing did not	Hepatitis A is a serious viral infection with fecal oral transmission,	90%–100% seropositivity rate	Not recommended for children younger than 1 y. Sensitivity to aluminum or		Available Worldwide Protective immunity 2–4 wk after receipt	Severe allergic reaction (eg, anaphylaxis) after a previous dose of any

(*continued on next page*)

Table 1
(continued)

Vaccine	Type	Administration	Booster Interval	Indications	Efficacy	Contraindications	Precautions	Comments	Side Effects
Station, NJ, USA)			seem to influence anamnestic immune response to the booster dose	which is the leading cause of vaccine-preventable illness occurring among nonimmune international travelers. The incidence rate can be as high as 20 cases/1000 travelers/mo during adventure or rural travel, and 3–6 cases/1000 travelers/mo in those going to tourist areas and resorts, in developing countries.		aluminum hydroxyl		of the first dose. Second dose confers lasting immunity for more than 10 y. Now included among routine immunizations in the United States for children Updated recommen-dations no longer call for dose IG when hepatitis A is given less than 2 wk before departure	hepatitis A–containing vaccine The most common adverse events are injection-site soreness and headache
HAV (AVAXIM; Sanofi Pasteur, Swiftwater, PA, USA)	Inactivated HAV, derived from GBM viral strain	IM deltoid, 2 doses	0 and 6–12 mo (delay in booster dose up to 66 mo in testing did not seem to influence anamnestic immune response to the booster dose	Hepatitis A is a serious viral infection with fecal oral transmission, which is the leading cause of vaccine-preventable illness occurring among non-immune international travelers. The incidence rate can be as high	90%–100% seropositivity rate	Not recommended for children younger than 1 y		Available in Europe Protective immunity 2–4 weeks after the receipt of first dose. Second dose confers lasting immunity for more than 10 y. Now included among routine immunizations in the United States for children	Severe allergic reaction (eg, anaphylaxis) after a previous dose of any hepatitis A–containing vaccine The most common adverse events are injection-site soreness and headache

				as 20 cases/1000 travelers/mo during adventure or rural travel, and 3–6 cases/1000 travelers/mo in those going to tourist areas and resorts, in developing countries.				Updated recommendations no longer call for dose IG when hepatitis A is given less than 2 wk before departure	
HAV (Epaxal Berna; Berna BioTech, Bern, Switzerland)	Inactivated virosomal HAV, derived from RG-SB viral strain	IM deltoid, 2 doses	0 and 6–12 mo (delay in booster dose up to 66 mo in testing did not seem to influence anamnestic immune response to the booster dose	Hepatitis A is a serious viral infection with fecal oral transmission, which is the leading cause of vaccine-preventable illness occurring among nonimmune international travelers. The incidence rate can be as high as 20 cases/1000 travelers/mo during adventure or rural travel, and 3–6 cases/1000 travelers/mo in those going to tourist areas and resorts, in	90%–100% seropositivity rate	Not recommended for children younger than 1 y		Available in Europe Protective immunity 2–4 wk after the receipt of first dose. Second dose confers lasting immunity for more than 10 y. Now included among routine immunizations in the United States for children Updated recommendations no longer call for dose IG when hepatitis A is given less than 2 wk before departure	Severe allergic reaction (eg, anaphylaxis) after a previous dose of any hepatitis A–containing vaccine The most common adverse events are injection-site soreness and headache

(continued on next page)

Table 1
(continued)

Vaccine	Type	Administration	Booster Interval	Indications	Efficacy	Contraindications	Precautions	Comments	Side Effects
				developing countries.					
Hepatitis B (HBV) (Engerix B; GlaxoSmith-Kline Biologicals, Pittsburgh, PA, USA)	Recom-binant HBV	IM deltoid, 3 doses	0, 1, and 6 mo (standard schedule) 0, 1, and 2 mo (accelerated schedule) Need for booster not determined	In many parts of Asia and Africa, up to 15% of the general population may be asymptomatic carriers of hepatitis B virus. Those who will live and work among the local population, and those who might have intimate contact or sexual contact with the local population, should consider immunization. Inadvertent exposures can occur during medical procedures and personal grooming/esthetic activities (shaving, manicures and pedicures, piercings, tattoos, etc)	90%–100% seropositivity rate			Included in the recommended childhood immunization schedule since 1990 In travelers at high risk, the possibility of nonsero-conversion among vaccine recipients should be considered. Risk factors include age more than 30 y, chronic medical conditions, smoking, obesity, male gender, and vaccine administration in buttock. Anti-HBs testing should be performed 1–6 mo after the last dose of vaccine. If no seroconversion has occurred, 1 additional dose of hepatitis B vaccine should be given and the titer rechecked 4–12 wk later. If no conversion has	Severe allergic reaction (eg, anaphylaxis) after a previous dose of any hepatitis B–containing vaccine or to any component of ENGERIX B, including yeast. The most common adverse events are injection-site soreness and tiredness.

								occurred, the second series is completed with 2 additional doses given at monthly intervals. Limited data from clinical studies show that titers and protection do not always correlate closely, even those with low or nondetectable titers may still be protected after immunization.	
HBV (Recombivax; Merck & Co, Inc, Whitehouse Station, NJ, USA)	Recombinant noninfectious subunit viral vaccine, derived from HBsAg produced in yeast cells	IM deltoid, 3 doses	0, 1, and 6 mo (standard schedule)	In many parts of Asia and Africa, up to 15% of the general population may be asymptomatic carriers of hepatitis B virus. Those who will live and work among the local population, and those who might have intimate contact or sexual contact with the local population, should consider immunization.	90%–100% seropositivity rate			Included in the recommended childhood immunization schedule since 1990. In travelers at high risk, the possibility of nonsero-conversion among vaccine recipients should be considered. Risk factors include age more than 30 y, chronic medical conditions, smoking, obesity, male gender, and vaccine	Severe allergic reaction (eg, anaphylaxis) after a previous dose of any hepatitis B–containing vaccine. The most common adverse events are injection-site soreness and tiredness.

(continued on next page)

Table 1
(continued)

Vaccine	Type	Administration	Booster Interval	Indications	Efficacy	Contraindications	Precautions	Comments	Side Effects
				Inadvertent exposures can occur during medical procedures and personal grooming/ esthetic activities (shaving, manicures and pedicures, piercings, tattoos, etc)				administration in buttock. Anti-HBs testing should be performed 1–6 mo after the last dose of vaccine. If no seroconversion has occurred, 1 additional dose of hepatitis B vaccine should be given and the titer rechecked 4–12 wk later. If no conversion has occurred, the second series is completed with 2 additional doses given at monthly intervals. Limited data from clinical studies show that titers and protection do not always correlate closely, even those with low or nondetectable titers may still be protected after immunization.	
Hepatitis A/B (Twinrix; GlaxoSmith-Kline	720 enzyme-linked immuno-sorbent assay units hepatitis	IM deltoid, 3 doses	0, 1, and 6 mo (standard schedule)	See above comments for hepatitis A and hepatitis B	100% seropositivity rate after first dose A, 82%			A pediatric formulation of the combined vaccine is not	Adverse reactions with Twinrix are similar to those

Biologicals, Pittsburgh, PA, USA)	A antigen and 20 μg hepatitis B antigen		0, 7, and 21–30 d (accelerated schedule) Need for booster not determined after standard schedule, a fourth dose is recommended 12 mo after the first dose to assure long-lasting immunity		after first dose B, 86% after second dose B, and 97% after third dose B			available in the United States but is available in other countries	experienced with the monovalent components. The most common adverse events are injection-site soreness, headache, and tiredness.
Immune globulin (IG)	Purified human IG	IM, deep Gluteus Maximus, 1 dose of 2 mL for 3-mo protection or 1 dose of 3 mL for 5-mo protection		Those unable to receive hepatitis A vaccination				Hepatitis A protection via passive transfer of preformed antibodies against hepatitis A (at least 100 IU/mL)	
Japanese encephalitis (JEV Vax, Biken; Sanofi Pasteur, Swiftwater, PA, USA)	Inactivated Japanese encephalitis virus (JEV) derived from infected mouse brains, with the final product containing less than 2 ng of myelin base protein per milliliter	Subcutaneous (SC), 3 doses	0, 7, and 30 d. Booster dose may be given after 2 y	Low risk of travel-associated JEV disease but high morbidity and mortality of disease. Not considered a risk for short-term travelers visiting usual tourist destinations in urban areas and developed resort areas. Visitors going to endemic rural areas during the transmission season face an estimated risk	88%–100% adults from nonendemic settings developed neutralizing antibodies after receiving 3 doses of vaccine	Not recommended for children younger than 1 y		Production was discontinued in 2006, but stockpiles of vaccine will be in use for children aged 1–16 y until depleted 2010/2011	Local pain, swelling, and redness at injection site in approximately 20% recipients. Systemic symptoms of fever, headache, and malaise in approximately 10% recipients. Hypersensitivity reactions, most commonly urticaria, angioedema, or both, in 15–62/10,000 vaccinated individuals

(*continued on next page*)

Table 1
(continued)

Vaccine	Type	Administration	Booster Interval	Indications	Efficacy	Contraindications	Precautions	Comments	Side Effects
				during a 1-mo period of 1:5000 or 1:20,000/wk. The risk of infection is decreased by personal protective measures to prevent mosquito bites. Japanese encephalitis has been acquired by short-term travelers to endemic rural areas, as such it should be offered to travelers going on trips of any length to rural areas during transmission season; travelers to an area of JEV outbreak; and expatriate workers, students, and missionaries who plan to travel, live, or work in urban, suburban, or farming communities in endemic areas.					almost immediately after or up to 2 wk after the first, second, or third dose of vaccine. The CDC recommends that vaccinated individuals be directly observed for 30 min after vaccine receipt and that they do not depart until 10 d after the last JEV dose.

Japanese encephalitis (JEV IXIARO; Intercel Biomedical, Livingston, UK, distributed by Novartis Vaccines, Cambridge, MA, USA)[47–49]	Inactivated, cell culture derived	IM, 0.5 mL, 2 doses	0 and 28 d. Approved on 2009, as such need for and timing of booster doses have not yet been determined		96% adults developed protective neutralizing antibodies	Not licensed in the United States for travelers younger than 17 y		Immunization should be completed at least 2 wk before traveling to endemic area. There are no data for the interchange-ability of JE vaccines or the use of IXIARO as a booster dose after a primary series with JE-VAX. It is currently recommended that those who previously received JE-VAX and require further vaccination should receive either a booster dose with JE-VAX or a primary series of 2 doses of IXIARO.	Contains protamine sulfate. The most common (≥10%) systemic adverse events were headache and myalgia. The most common (≥10%) injection-site reactions were pain and tenderness. Safety and effectiveness have not been established in pregnant women and nursing mothers.
Meningococcus (A/C/Y/W-135) (MCV4) (Menactra; Sanofi Pasteur, Swiftwater, PA, USA)	A, C, Y, W135 polysaccharides conjugated to diphtheria toxin protein	IM, 1 dose	Booster interval has not been determined, with estimated protective immunity lasting 7 y or more. Individuals who received the MPSV4 vaccine in the past can be boosted with MCV4 if	[a]Due to outbreaks of meningococcal disease among Hajj pilgrims with secondary spread to family and friends after the pilgrims returned home, Saudi Arabia mandated vaccine		Licensed for use among individuals aged 11–55 y		The Advisory Committee on Immunization Practices routinely recommends vaccination with quadrivalent meningococcal conjugate vaccine for individuals 11–18 y old and	The most frequently reported adverse effects reported with MCV4 (Menactra) in children 2–10 y of age were local effects at the injection site (eg, pain) and irritability. Diarrhea,

(continued on next page)

Table 1
(continued)

Vaccine	Type	Administration	Booster Interval	Indications	Efficacy	Contraindications	Precautions	Comments	Side Effects
			they remain at risk for exposure	requirement in 2003 for all persons traveling to Saudi Arabia during the annual Hajj, and either quadrivalent vaccine will fulfill the requirement. In some countries, bivalent meningococcal polysaccharide vaccine or conjugate vaccines vs A and C are commonly available; however, outbreaks involving Y and W-135 have occurred during some Hajj outbreaks. Vaccine is also recommended for travelers going to live or work in certain areas of South America and sub-Saharan Africa and other areas where meningococcal disease is epidemic or				incoming college freshman who will live in large residence halls on campus. Some colleges require vaccination before matriculation. It is also recommended for individuals at increased risk for disease, including microbiologists routinely exposed to strains, military recruits, individuals with terminal complement component deficiencies, and persons with anatomic or functional asplenia. Enables enhanced immunity through activation of a strong T-cell response	drowsiness, and anorexia were also common in this age group. The most common adverse effects reported with MCV4 (Menactra) in adolescents and adults 11–55 y of age were local effects at the site of injection (eg, pain), headache, and fatigue. In the clinical studies comparing safety and efficacy of MCV4 (Menactra) and MPSV4 (Menomune), adverse local effects were reported more frequently with MCV4 (Menactra) than with MPSV4 (Menomune); however, the incidence of systemic adverse effects reported with the conjugated vaccine was

				hyperendemic among the local residents.	similar to that reported with the unconjugated vaccine.
Meningococcus (A/C/Y/W-135) (MPSV4) (Menimmune; Sanofi Pasteur, Swiftwater, PA, USA)	Polysaccharide vaccine	SC, 1 dose	Estimated protective interval 3–5 y A second dose is recommended after 2–3 y in children living in high-risk areas who received their first dose at younger than 4 y	Due to outbreaks of meningococcal disease among Hajj pilgrims with secondary spread to family and friends after the pilgrims returned home, Saudi Arabia mandated vaccine requirement in 2003 for all persons traveling to Saudi Arabia during the annual Hajj, and either quadrivalent vaccine will fulfill the requirement. In some countries, bivalent meningococcal polysaccharide vaccine or conjugate vaccines vs A and C are commonly available; however, outbreaks involving Y and W-135 have occurred	The most frequently reported adverse effects reported with MCV4 (Menactra) in children 2–10 y of age were local effects at the injection site (eg, pain) and irritability. Diarrhea, drowsiness, and anorexia were also common in this age group. The most common adverse effects reported with MCV4 (Menactra) in adolescents and adults 11–55 y of age were local effects at the site of injection (eg, pain), headache, and fatigue. In the clinical studies comparing safety and efficacy of MCV4 (Menactra) and MPSV4 (Menomune), adverse local

(continued on next page)

Table 1
(continued)

Vaccine	Type	Administration	Booster Interval	Indications	Efficacy	Contraindications	Precautions	Comments	Side Effects
				during some Hajj outbreaks. Vaccine is also recommended for travelers going to live or work in certain areas of South America and sub-Saharan Africa and other areas where meningococcal disease is epidemic or hyperendemic among the local residents.					effects were reported more frequently with MCV4 (Menactra) than with MPSV4 (Menomune); however, the incidence of systemic adverse effects reported with the conjugated vaccine was similar to that reported with the unconjugated vaccine.
Plague	Killed bacterial vaccine	IM, 1 mL, 3 doses	0, 1, and 4–7 mo Boost if risk exposure persists. First 2 booster doses (0.1–0.2 mL) 6 mo apart, then 1 booster dose at 1- to 2-y intervals	International travelers going on standard tourist itineraries to countries of Asia, Africa, and the Americas where plague is reported unlikely to be at risk. Those at high risk include field biologists and those who will reside or work in areas where avoidance of rodents and fleas is difficult.	Poorly documented protective effect	Not commercially available			Pain, redness, and induration at the site of injections. Systemic symptoms include headache, fever, and malaise after repeated doses.

Rabies (HDCV) (HDCV Imovax; Sanofi Pasteur, Swiftwater, PA, USA) or rabies vaccine absorbed (RVA; GlaxoSmith-Kline Biologicals, Pittsburgh, PA, USA) or purified chick embryo vaccine (PCEC) (RabAvert; Chiron, Emeryville, CA, USA)	Inactivated virus vaccine. RVA and PCEC are derived from virus grown in tissue culture cells in a medium clear of human albumin.	IM, 1 mL, 3 doses	0, 7, and 21 or 28 d Boost after 2 years if continued risk of exposure or test serum antibody level	Animal bites, especially dog bites, present a potential rabies hazard to those who travel to urban and rural areas in Central and South America, the Middle East, Africa and Asia. Preexposure rabies immunization is recommended for rural travelers, especially adventure travelers, who go to remote areas, and for expatriate workers, missionaries, and their families living in countries where rabies is a recognized risk. Preexposure prophylaxis simplifies the postbite medical care of a person following an exposure in a high-risk area.		The 3 vaccine products may be used inter-changeably in preexposure rabies immunization given IM. RVA and PCEC vaccines may only be given IM.	Mild local reactions are common, including erythema, pain, and swelling at the injection site. Mild systemic symptoms including headache, dizziness, nausea, abdominal pain, and myalgias may develop in some recipients. In approximately 5% of individuals receiving booster doses of HDCV for preexposure prophylaxis, a serum sickness–like illness characterized by urticaria, fever, malaise, arthralgias, arthritis, nausea, and vomiting may develop 2–21 d after the vaccine dose is administered.

(continued on next page)

Table 1
(continued)

Vaccine	Type	Administration	Booster Interval	Indications	Efficacy	Contraindications	Precautions	Comments	Side Effects
Rabies (HDCV), Imovax intradermal administration	Inactivated virus vaccine	Intradermal, 0.1 mL, 3 doses	0, 7, and 21 or 28 d Boost after 2 years if continued risk of exposure or test serum antibody level	Animal bites, especially dog bites, present a potential rabies hazard to those who travel to urban and rural areas in Central and South America, the Middle East, Africa, and Asia. Preexposure rabies immunization is recommended for rural travelers, especially adventure travelers, who go to remote areas, and for expatriate workers, missionaries, and their families living in countries where rabies is a recognized risk. Preexposure prophylaxis simplifies the postbite medical care of a person following an exposure in a high-risk area.				The efficacy of the intradermal vaccine series is compromised if chloroquine prophylaxis against malaria is started within 3 wk after the third dose of intradermal vaccine.	

Tick borne encephalitis (Encepur; Chiron, Behring, Germany), standard schedule	IM, 3 doses	0, 28, and 300 d Boost 3 years after last dose	Tick borne encephalitis is caused by infection with either Central European encephalitis virus (CEEV) in Europe or Russian Spring Summer encephalitis virus (RSSEV) in the Common-wealth of Independent States, transmitted by Ixodes ticks in endemic areas from April through August or ingestion of unpasteurized dairy products from infected cows, goats, or sheep.		Vaccination is currently not available in the United States Vaccines are interchangeable Because vaccine is not available in the United States, travelers will need to rely on personal protective measures against insect exposure, including protective clothing, DEET on all exposed areas of skin, and treating outdoor clothing with permethrin-containing insecticide. All travelers to these areas are advised not to eat unpasteurized dairy products.
Tick borne encephalitis (Encepur; Chiron, Behring, Germany), rapid schedule	SC, 3 doses	0,7, and 21 d First booster dose at 15 mo after first vaccine dose, second booster dose at 36 mo after the first booster	Tick borne encephalitis is caused by infection with either CEEV in Europe or RSSEV in the Common-wealth of Independent States, transmitted by Ixodes ticks in endemic areas from April through		Vaccination is currently not available in the United States Vaccines are interchangeable Because vaccine is not available in the United States, travelers will need to rely on personal protective measures against insect exposure, including protective clothing, DEET on all exposed areas of skin, and

(*continued on next page*)

Table 1
(continued)

Vaccine	Type	Administration	Booster Interval	Indications	Efficacy	Contraindications	Precautions	Comments	Side Effects
				August or ingestion of unpasteurized dairy products from infected cows, goats, or sheep.			treating outdoor clothing with permethrin-containing insecticide. All travelers to these areas are advised not to eat unpasteurized dairy products.		
Tick borne encephalitis (FSME; Immuno, Vienna, Austria), standard schedule	Chick embryo cell cultures	SC, 3 doses	0, 1–3, and 9–12 mo after dose 2 Boost 3 years after last dose	Tick borne encephalitis is caused by infection with either CEEV in Europe or RSSEV in the Common-wealth of Independent States, transmitted by Ixodes ticks in endemic areas from April through August or ingestion of unpasteurized dairy products from infected cows, goats, or sheep.			Available in Canada and Europe Vaccination is currently not available in the United States Vaccines are interchangeable Because vaccine is not available in the United States, travelers will need to rely on personal protective measures against insect exposure, including protective clothing, DEET on all exposed areas of skin, and treating outdoor clothing with permethrin-containing insecticide. All travelers to these areas are advised not to eat unpasteurized dairy products.		
Tick borne encephalitis (FSME; Immuno, Vienna,	Chick embryo cell cultures	SC, 3 doses	First booster dose at 15 mo after the first vaccine dose, second booster at	Tick borne encephalitis is caused by infection with either CEEV in Europe or			Vaccination is currently not available in the United States Vaccines are interchangeable		

Austria), rapid schedule			36 mo after the first booster	RSSEV in the Common-wealth of Independent States, transmitted by Ixodes ticks in endemic areas from April through August or ingestion of unpasteurized dairy products from infected cows, goats, or sheep.		Because vaccine is not available in the United States, travelers will need to rely on personal protective measures against insect exposure, including protective clothing, DEET on all exposed areas of skin, and treating outdoor clothing with permethrin-containing insecticide. All travelers to these areas are advised not to eat unpasteurized dairy products.	
Typhoid (Typhim Vi; Sanofi Pasteur, Swiftwater, PA, USA)	Highly purified Vi capsular polysaccharide	IM, 1 dose	Boost after 2 y for continued risk of exposure	The incidence of typhoid in American travelers is relatively low (50–170 cases/1 million travelers), but among reported cases in the United States, 62% were acquired during international travel. Particularly, high risk is experienced in travel to Mexico, Peru, India, Pakistan, and Chile. Southeast Asia	Children older than 2 y Discard vaccine dose if discolored or particulate material is present	Elicits immunity 10 d after receipt of a single primary dose The protection against typhoid fever from immunization can be overwhelmed by ingestion of highly contaminated food.	Generally well tolerated. The following adverse effects were reported: common and generally mild, constipation, abdominal cramps, diarrhea, nausea, vomiting, anorexia, fever, headache, and urticarial rash. Very rarely dermatitis, pruritis and urticaria, anaphylaxis, paresthesias, and arthralgias and myalgias.

(*continued on next page*)

Table 1
(continued)

Vaccine	Type	Administration	Booster Interval	Indications	Efficacy	Contraindications	Precautions	Comments	Side Effects
				and sub-Saharan Africa are also considered areas of increased risk. Travelers to high-risk areas who will be staying for more than 1 mo.					
Typhoid (Vivotif; Berna BioTech, Bern, Switzerland)	Live attenuated strain of Salmonella typhi bacteria (Ty21A)	Oral, 4 doses	1 capsule orally on empty stomach every 2 d. Booster at 5 y with another 4-capsule regimen A liquid suspension form is available in Europe		43%–96% in field trials in residents of endemic areas	Children older than 6 y Safety in immune-compromised individuals has not yet been demonstrated, and this vaccine should not be administered to them. The vaccine is not recommended for pregnant women	The protection against typhoid fever from immunization can be overwhelmed by ingestion of highly contaminated food.	Any condition that interferes with virus strain multiplication in the bowel may result in an insufficient antigen stimulus to induce an adequate protective response. It should not be administered during an acute gastrointestinal illness or if the individual is receiving antibiotics active against salmonella. Proguanil, one component of Malarone used for malaria prevention and treatment,	The following adverse effects were reported: common and generally mild, constipation, abdominal cramps, diarrhea, nausea, vomiting, anorexia, fever, headache, and urticarial rash. Very rarely dermatitis, pruritis and urticaria, anaphylaxis, paresthesias, and arthralgias and myalgias.

								decreases the immune response to typhoid vaccine, as such they should be administered 10 or more days after the final dose of vaccine.	
Yellow Fever (YF Vax; Sanofi Pasteur, Swiftwater, PA, USA)[48]	Live attenuated vaccine prepared from the 17D strain of yellow fever virus in eggs. Vaccine production is controlled by the WHO.	SC, 1 dose	Booster every 10 y, although immunity is possibly lifelong	Immunization is required for entry into some countries within the endemic zones in sub-Saharan Africa or tropical South America or may be recommended to travelers either going to rural tropical areas within the endemic zones or to both rural and urban areas during yellow fever outbreaks.	Seroconversion rates of 95% or more and a protection rate of more than 99% in immuno-competent individuals	The vaccine is not recommended for individuals with a history of anaphylaxis to eggs Immuno-suppression is a contra-indication to receiving the vaccine Most travel experts would consider administering yellow fever vaccine to HIV-positive travelers if the CD4 count is greater than 400 Not for children younger than 6 mo because of a significant but rare (1/8 million doses) risk of vaccine-associated neurotropic		A list of countries requiring yellow fever vaccination for entry can be found on either the CDC or WHO Websites. If a person for whom the vaccine is contraindicated must travel to one of these countries, a signed statement by a licensed vaccination center, on letterhead stationary, that states that yellow fever vaccine could not be administered to the traveler because medical contra-indications will be accepted	Between 1996 and 2002, 13 cases of yellow fever vaccine–associated viscerotropic disease (YEL-AVD) were reported by the CDC and WHO. It occurred 2–5 d after receiving vaccine and was a febrile illness, which led to multiple organ failure. YEL-AVD is likely related to transient viremia that occurs after vaccine receipt, and the risk is considered to be rare in first-time vaccine recipients. Risk increases with age (3.5/100,000

(*continued on next page*)

Table 1
(continued)

Vaccine	Type	Administration	Booster Interval	Indications	Efficacy	Contraindications	Precautions	Comments	Side Effects
						disease (YEL-AND) Children 6–9 mo of age should not be vaccinated unless traveling to an area with an outbreak Generally not recommended in pregnancy except when travel to a highly endemic area cannot be avoided and the risk of actual disease is thought to be greater than the theoretical risk of adverse vaccine effects		instead of the vaccination statement according to WHO regulations.	vaccine recipients aged 65–74 y and 9.1/100,000 vaccine recipients older than 75 y). However, the protection afforded by the vaccine probably outweighs risk in those senior citizens who are traveling to endemic regions.
Polio (IPV; Sanofi Pasteur, Swiftwater, PA, USA)	Inactivated	SC, 0.5 mL deltoid. Adults who are traveling to areas where WPV cases are still occurring and who are unvaccinated, incompletely vaccinated, or whose vaccination status is unknown	For adults, available data do not indicate the need for more than 1 lifetime booster dose with IPV	Because of polio eradication efforts, the number of countries where travelers are at risk for polio (WPV) has decreased dramatically over the last 30 y, and most of the global population live		The minimum age for IPV vaccination is 6 wks IPV should not be administered to individuals who have experienced a severe allergic reaction (anaphylaxis) after a previous dose of IPV or		OPV is no longer recommended for routine immunization in the United States	Minor local reactions can follow IPV. No serious reactions have been documented.

	should receive 2 doses of IPV at least 4 wk apart and a third dose should be administered 6–12 mo after the second dose. If there is inadequate time before travel and fewer than 3 doses are administered, the remaining doses to complete a 3-dose series should be administered when feasible. Adults who are traveling to areas where poliomyelitis cases are occurring and who have received a primary series with either OPV or IPV in childhood should receive another dose of IPV before departure.	in areas considered free of WPV circulation, including the Western Hemisphere; the Western Pacific region, including China; and the European region. Vaccination is recommended for all travelers to polio-endemic or -epidemic areas, including countries with recent proven WPV circulation and neighboring countries. As of September 2008, these areas include some but not all countries in Africa, South Asia, Southeast Asia, and the Middle East.	after receiving streptomycin, polymixin B, or neomycin because these are contained in trace amounts in the vaccine.	

(continued on next page)

Table 1
(continued)

Vaccine	Type	Administration	Booster Interval	Indications	Efficacy	Contraindications	Precautions	Comments	Side Effects
Smallpox	Vaccinia virus					No longer available commercially. It is available on a case-by-case basis from the CDC based on individual review. The requirement for smallpox vaccination for international travel was removed from the WHO regulations in 1982. The last case of smallpox acquired via natural transmission was reported in 1977.			

Required vaccination before travel

Yellow fever is the only vaccine currently required by international health regulations for travel to and from certain countries in tropical South America and sub-Saharan Africa. Updated lists of *Yellow Fever Vaccination Certification Requirements by Country* and *Authorized U.S. Yellow Fever Vaccination Clinics* are found on the CDC Traveler's Health Web site (www.cdc.gov/travel/content/vaccinations.aspx).

Over the last several years, quadrivalent (A/C/Y/W-135) meningococcal vaccination, which must have been issued not more than 3 years and not less than 10 days before arrival, has been required by the Saudi Arabian government for all infants, children, and adult pilgrims for annual travel during the Hajj. The immunization status is checked before issuance of a visa, which is not issued unless documented compliance is provided. A travel health provider letter may be issued to those individuals who are unable to receive vaccine; however, this does not guarantee issuance of a visa for Hajj travel.

MALARIA AND DENGUE PREVENTION AND THE CURRENT STATUS OF VACCINE DEVELOPMENT

Malaria in humans is caused by 5 species of the protozoan genus *Plasmodium*: *P falciparum*, *P vivax*, *P ovale* (recently split into 2 subspecies), *P malariae*, and most recently and much less frequently *P knowlesi*. Malaria is primarily transmitted by the bite of infected female *Anopheles* mosquitoes, although transmission is also documented via blood transfusion, organ transplantation, and needle sharing. *Anopheles* spp are evening feeders; therefore, transmission occurs primarily from dusk to dawn. Annually, malaria causes 350 to 500 million infections and 1 million deaths globally, largely affecting children in areas of Central and South America, parts of the Caribbean, Eastern Europe, Asia, Africa, and Oceania (see **Fig. 1** for a map of at-risk areas for malaria transmission. Regularly updated maps are available on the WHO and CDC Websites [www.cdc.gov/malaria/map/index.html]). Thirty thousand travelers from Europe and North America contract malaria each year, with 10,745 cases reported in US residents to the CDC from 1997 to 2006. Of the reported cases in the United States, 59.3% were acquired in sub-Saharan Africa, 13.9% in Asia, 13.3% in the Caribbean and Central and South America, and 0.03% in Oceania. However, when considered in the context of volume of travel to these locations, the regions of highest estimated relative risk are West Africa and Oceania; other parts of Africa, South Asia, and South America are felt to have moderate risk, whereas,

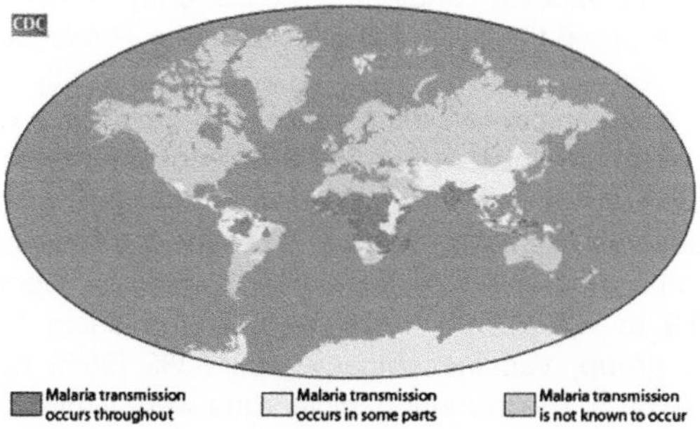

Fig. 1. Malaria transmission zones. (*Courtesy of* the US Centers for Disease Control and Prevention. A regularly updated map can be found at http://www.cdc.gov/malaria/about/distribution.html.)

portions of Central America and other parts of Asia are of relatively lower risk. Individual traveler risk varies substantially by region, including areas of differing altitude, urban versus rural travel, by season, and between travelers.[24] The level of risk presented by a particular itinerary decides whether it may be appropriate to recommend mosquito avoidance methods only, mosquito avoidance methods and chemoprophylaxis, or no specific interventions. Even short exposure, such as that experienced by cruise ship passengers, may pose risk in an area of intense transmission.

Malaria chemoprophylaxis is a dynamic topic, because the risk of transmission is influenced by an individual travelers' behavior, may not be uniformly distributed in individual countries, and is affected by changes in resistance patterns and the availability and usefulness of newer and older drugs. The highest-risk travelers are those first- or second-generation immigrants currently living in nonendemic countries who return to their countries of origin to VFRs.[23–25] These individuals often consider themselves not at risk because they grew up in an endemic area and believe themselves immune. Unfortunately, acquired immunity is lost very quickly on leaving an endemic area. Several options for malaria chemoprophylaxis are currently available, and no single regimen is ideal for all travelers. A thorough discussion of vector avoidance, malaria chemoprophylaxis, and treatment may be found elsewhere.

Malaria vaccination development has faced numerous challenges since the initial cloning of malaria antigens in the early 1980s. At present, several questions remain regarding vaccine mode of action in this parasite's complex and incompletely understood infection biology, efficacy, dosage schedules, and potential duration of effect. Resources for research funding are relatively scarce. Goals of vaccine development have been to either prevent blood-stage infection completely via destruction of sporozoites before they enter the liver or kill the infected hepatocytes (preerythrocytic vaccine) or to limit parasite growth and density in the blood compartment via destruction of the infected erythrocytes (blood-stage vaccine), with the goal of providing a durable immune response similar in efficacy to that induced by natural infection. Significant antigenic diversity has been a barrier to the development of immunity in both the preerythrocytic and blood stages of parasite development. Although immunity to severe life-threatening disease is evidently acquired early in childhood in areas of intense malaria transmission, clearly demonstrating clinical immunity, vaccine trials have been limited by the lack of an immunologic correlate of effectiveness in vaccinated individuals.[26,27] An ideal vaccine should be directed against several novel antigens, perhaps T-cell targets, expressed in several stages of parasite development, that are likely to be highly conserved in sequence and robustly recognized by vaccine-induced immune response.[28,29]

Several stage-specific vaccine candidates are currently in trials to prevent *P falciparum* infection. One preerythrocytic vaccine targeting *P falciparum* circumsporozoite protein, GlaxoSmithKline RTS, S/AS02$_D$, is currently in phase 3 trial (NCT00866619) in 11 African centers with results expected at the end of 2011. Phase 1/2b trial of this vaccine administered to 214 Mozambican infants at 10, 14, and 18 weeks of age, staggered with routine vaccines, reported a good safety profile (32.7% vs 31.8% serious adverse events in the control group) and remained somewhat efficacious at 14 months (geometric mean titers of anticircumsporozoite antibodies declined from 199.9 to 7.3 EU/mL at 12 months, remaining 15-fold higher than that of the control group, vaccine efficacy was 33% [95% confidence interval: −4.3 to 56.9, $P = .076$]).[30] The immunogenicity data were similar to those previously reported in older children and adults.[30,31] No relation between anticircumsporozoite antibody titer and protection was demonstrated in Mozambican children aged 1 to 4 years.[31]

To successfully affect global malaria elimination, it is also crucial to attack other major malarial species that affect humans. Vaccine progress against *P vivax*, a cause of significant morbidity and mortality in Central and South America, the eastern Mediterranean, and Asia, with an estimated 70 million to 391 million cases annually, is not nearly as advanced.[32]

Dengue, currently the most prevalent arthropod-borne viral illness in humans, is caused by 4 serotypes of the dengue virus (DENV). Dengue is a member of the Flaviviridae family, as are yellow fever and Japanese encephalitis. DENVs are transmitted to humans via the bite of peridomestic day-biting *Aedes* mosquitoes, most prominently *Aedes aegypti*. Infection with DENV causes a spectrum of clinical illness, ranging from a usually mild, acute self-limited febrile illness, dengue fever, to life-threatening hemorrhagic and capillary leak syndromes of dengue hemorrhagic fever/dengue shock syndrome (DHF/DSS). DENV causes an estimated 25 million to 100 million cases of dengue fever and 250,000 cases of DHF yearly worldwide. 2.5 billion people are estimated to be at risk for infection (**Fig. 2**, a world map indicating regions with known risk of dengue is available at http://www.cdc.gov/ncidod/dvbid/dengue). The United States has witnessed the return of autochthonous transmission since 1980, initially described in Texas, but now reported in Hawaii, Florida, and Puerto Rico. Geosentinel data, collected on 6 continents, showed dengue fever to be the second most common cause of systemic febrile illness, excluding diarrheal diseases, in returning travelers and the most common cause in travelers returning from the Caribbean, South America, Southeast Asia, and South Central Asia.[15]

In brief, the pathogenesis of DHF/DSS reflects a complex interaction of viral virulence determinants and the host immune system. Infection with one serotype of DENV renders the individual immune to that strain for life but with only transient immunity to other strains, and individuals are at risk for DHF/DSS with secondary DENV infection with another strain. An increased risk of DHF/DSS also occurs in children within their first year of life when born to DENV-immune mothers. These observations served as the basis for the hypothesis of antibody-dependent immune enhancement (ADE) in DHF/DSS, which is supported by the findings of increased peak viremia in severe DHF/DSS, and ADE is seen in vitro in DENV-infected monocytes. A pathologic cytokine response, including increased levels of interferon γ, interleukin 10, and tumor necrosis factor γ, after $CD8^+$ cell activation is thought to contribute to the capillary leak syndrome seen with dengue hemorrhagic fever (DHF). Most protective antibodies are directed against the surface E glycoprotein of the virus. Antibodies to the M and NS1 proteins also have been shown to demonstrate some protection. At present, there is no established dengue immune correlate of infection.

Dengue vaccine development dates back to the 1920s. At present, no DENV vaccine is approved by the US Food and Drug Administration. Vaccine development

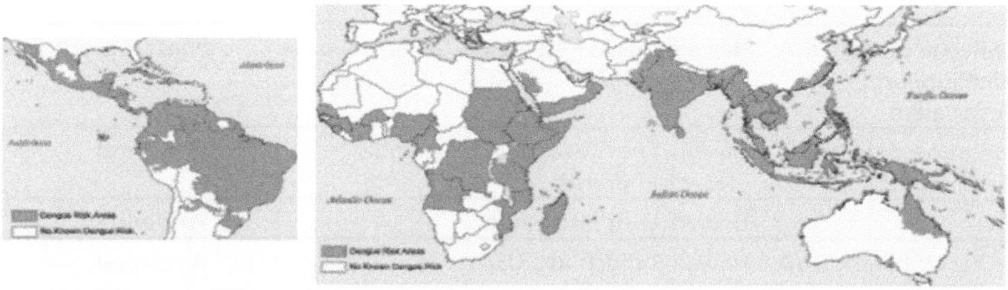

Fig. 2. Dengue transmission zones. (*Courtesy of* the US Centers for Disease Control and Prevention. A regularly updated interactive map can be found at http://www.healthmap.org/dengue/index.phpt.)

has been hampered by the absence of a validated animal model of dengue infection. Based on the current understanding of virus-immune system interactions, an effective vaccine should produce high titers of neutralizing antibodies against all 4 strains. Failure to achieve this potentially increases the individual's risk of severe DHF/DSS if challenged by a natural virus infection with a different strain. Several tetravalent live attenuated virus candidate vaccines are in development (see **Table 2** for a list of current candidate DENV vaccines). Tetravalent serologic responses have been observed in some individuals during trials; whereas each portion of the tetravalent vaccines has not been shown to elicit high titer responses, monovalent vaccines were shown to elicit higher levels of neutralizing antibodies than when they were combined in multivalent combinations, and many individuals mount insufficient levels of neutralizing antibodies despite multiple immunizations. Alternative vaccine candidates include subunit-based vaccines containing purified proteins or DNA plasmids, which have been shown to produce protective antibodies in mice at fairly low neutralizing titers; live attenuated vaccines, including dengue and dengue-yellow fever chimeras; and nonreplicating vaccines, including virus-like particles, DNA vaccines, and inactivated virus vaccines. Long-lasting protective neutralizing antibodies are elicited against a specific serotype, but they have been shown to be poorly cross-reactive against infection with another serotype. Similar problems were encountered in the development of OPV, and the imbalance in seroconversion was overcome by the administration of 3 doses of the multivalent vaccine.[33–38] A Sanofi Pasteur

Table 2
Current status of dengue virus vaccine development

Vaccine Type	Developer	Collaborator	Status
Live Attenuated Virus, Tetravalent	Walter Reed Army Institute of Research, USA	GlaxoSmithKline	Phase 2
Live Attenuated Virus, Tetravalent	National Institutes of Health, USA	Biologic E. Panacea	Phase 2
Live Attenuated Virus, Tetravalent	Mahidol University, Thailand	Sanofi Pasteur	Completed phase 2, halted
Live Attenuated Virus, Tetravalent	National Institute for Allergy & Infectious Disease, USA	Vabiotech	Phase 1/2
Live Chimeric Virus, Tetravalent	CDC, USA	Inviragen	Phase 1
Live Chimeric Virus, Tetravalent	Acambis, USA (acquired by Sanofi Pasteur, 2008)	Sanofi Pasteur	Phase 3
Live Recombinant DNA and Subunit, Tetravalent	Naval Medical Research Center, USA	University of Pittsburgh	Phase 1/preclinical
Replication-defective Arbovirus (E)	University of Texas Medical Branch	Acambis	Preclinical
DNA	University of Pittsburgh		Preclinical
Live Recombinant DNA and Subunit, Tetravalent	Hawaii Biotech Inc, USA		Preclinical

Data from Refs.[35–38]

tetravalent live attenuated chimeric yellow fever-dengue vaccine has entered hase 3 trials (NCT01134263). Phase 2 trials suggest that the vaccine is safe and immunogenic.[35] Preliminary results of an ongoing phase 2b efficacy and safety trial in Thai children are expected to be available by the end of 2012.

TRAVELER'S DIARRHEA AND THE ROLE OF VACCINATION

Traveler's diarrhea is a significant concern among international travelers. It is usually self-limited, consisting of several days of watery diarrhea, sometimes accompanied by low-grade fever, headache, malaise, nausea, and abdominal cramping. Thirty to seventy percent of travelers may be affected during a 2-week trip, largely depending on the travel destination. The highest attack rates are seen in travelers to Asia, Africa, Mexico, Latin America, and the Middle East. Intermediate risk is seen with travel to the Caribbean, Eastern Europe, the former Soviet States, southern Europe, Israel, and South Africa. Travel to the developed nations in North America, Europe, Japan, New Zealand, and Australia provides the lowest attack rates.[39,40] A recent study examining the Geosentinel data found that female travelers seem to be at disproportionately increased risk for acute diarrhea, chronic diarrhea, and irritable bowel syndrome than male travelers.[41] Contrary to popular belief, traveler's diarrhea does not only occur in travelers from temperate, economically developed countries to semitropical and tropical developing countries, as evidenced by the serious recent outbreak of shiga-toxin–producing *Escherichia coli* serogroup O104:H4 (STEC) with hemolytic uremic syndrome (HUS) in northern Germany. Any traveler may experience an acute intestinal upset, as this is increasingly recognized as a disturbance of the normal ecology of an individual's gastrointestinal tract by exposures to new water, foods, and spices as well as to microorganisms. Gastrointestinal dysfunction, in the form of irritable bowel syndrome, may persist in up to 13% of individuals who develop traveler's diarrhea.[42,43] Other postinfectious sequelae include Guillain-Barre and reactive arthritis.

Many viral, bacterial, and protozoal microorganisms cause traveler's diarrhea. Symptoms may result from the ingestion of preformed toxins, such as that seen with *Bacillus cereus*, staphylococcal food poisoning, and botulism. In general, bacteria are the most commonly identified cause of acute diarrheal disease in travelers visiting tropical and developing countries (80%–90%), with risk modified by geographic region, time of year, and the presence of local outbreaks. In many cases, no causative organism may be identified. Enterotoxigenic strains of *E coli* (ETEC), which may carry both heat-labile and heat-stable plasmid-coded enterotoxins, are the most commonly identified bacterial cause. Oral cholera vaccine produces some protection against traveler's diarrhea, because it elicits antibody production against the B subunit of cholera toxin, which cross-reacts with the heat-labile toxin of ETEC. In the past decade, *Campylobacter* species, most commonly *Campylobacter jejuni*, have become increasingly common pathogenic agents of traveler's diarrhea. These seem to have seasonal and geographic variance, with the peak incidence in the United States in summer months, whereas the peak incidence in other regions, such as North Africa, occurs in winter months. Other bacteria implicated in traveler's diarrhea include enteroadherent *E coli*; *Salmonella* spp, including *S typhi*; *Shigella* spp; *Yersinia enterocolitica*; *Aeromonas*; *Vibrio* spp, including *V parahemolyticus*, *V cholera*, and *V vulnificus*; and *Plesiomonas shigelloides*. Norovirus is a common cause of traveler's diarrhea (10%–15% cases), notably in several cruise-ship outbreaks. Rotavirus and astroviruses are less common pathogens in adults (5%–14%). Hepatitis A and E also cause gastrointestinal illness in travelers. Hepatitis E is of particular concern in pregnant women as it may lead to severe, life-threatening illness. Most parasites implicated in traveler's diarrhea are protozoa, including *Giardia lamblia*, and less commonly *Cryptosporidium* spp, *Cyclospora cayetenensis*, *Isospora belli*, *Entamoeba histolytica*, and occasionally *Dientamoeba fragilis*. Helminths are also reported to cause diarrheal disease in travelers. Ingested plant, fish, and shellfish toxin-related illness, including Ackee poisoning, Scombroid, Ciguatera, paralytic, neurotoxic, and diarrheal shellfish poisonings, may also cause gastrointestinal disease in travelers.

Pretravel vaccination and counseling regarding safe food and water practices can provide varying degrees of protection against enteric infection; however, even with the greatest of care, the risk of developing diarrhea remains high. The natural protective mechanisms of the intestinal tract, most prominently gastric acidity, and immune stimulation provided by vaccination can be overwhelmed by the ingestion of heavily contaminated water and food and moderated by traveler specifics, such as immune suppression, hypochlorhydria, gastrectomy, and concurrent medications.[44] Environments lacking appropriate sanitary conditions and clean water provide significant stool contamination highly accessible to flies. Attempts to select safe foods, such as those freshly prepared and served hot, can be counteracted by contamination introduced during preparation, storage, and handling.[45]

Although many travelers want to experience local culture and cuisine, commonsense food and water precautions may help individuals to make safer choices. These precautions are harder to maintain in those VFRs, those staying in local homes or pursuing more adventurous travel, and those staying in highly contaminated areas for prolonged periods of time. This article does not focus on a detailed discussion of food and water precautions, water treatment, and treatment and prevention of traveler's diarrhea.

At present, few vaccines are available to prevent the most common causes of traveler's diarrhea. Hepatitis A vaccine and oral and intramuscular typhoid vaccines are effective and well tolerated, although limited data address the actual level of protection afforded by oral and injectable typhoid vaccines to travelers from nonendemic areas visiting endemic areas.[46] Cholera vaccine seems moderately effective against non-O139 strains. A transcutaneous *E coli* LT vaccine is currently in phase 3 trials.

GENERAL RECOMMENDATIONS

Additional pretravel recommendations, such as jet lag mitigation, protection against sun exposure, venous thrombosis avoidance, prevention and treatment of altitude illness, baric risk, marine bites and envenomation attendant to diving and water sports, and the risks of extreme heat or cold, depend on the individual traveler's agenda. Safety regulations and practices are less prevalent in many nations than in the United States, Canada, and Europe. Most US medical insurance policies do not provide coverage for illness or accidents occurring outside the country and coverage for medical evacuation; however, many companies provide this insurance. A thoughtful discussion of these topics, and the management of the traveler returning with illness, lies outside the scope of this article.

In summary, individual travel for business and pleasure has grown tremendously in the past several decades, with an increasing number of at-risk individuals traveling and travelers visiting more remote and dangerous areas. Travelers potentially face several risks during travel. Thorough, epidemiologically and itinerary-based discussion and management of these risks before travel with a provider appropriately educated and experienced to provide this care, taking into consideration the individuals' risk tolerance, medical belief system, and finances, provide individuals the ability to travel more safely and to maximally experience their trip. Information gleaned from illness and injury experienced by travelers and, infections developed during travel and potentially brought back to the home country, continues to improve care and inform home countries about potential risks to their citizens and to improve the global management of transmissible illness.

REFERENCES

1. Hamer DH, Connor BA. Travel health knowledge, attitudes and practices among United States travelers. J Travel Med 2004;11:23–6.
2. Toovey S, Jamieson A, Holloway M. Traveler's knowledge, attitudes and practices on the prevention of infectious diseases: results from a study at Johannesburg International Airport. J Travel Med 2004;11:16–22.
3. Smith AD, Bradley DJ, Smith V, et al. Imported malaria and high-risk groups: observational study using UK surveillance data 1987-2006. BMJ 2008;337:a120.
4. Steffen R, Amitirigala I, Mutsch M. Health risks among travelers—need for regular updates. J Travel Med 2008;15(3):145–6.
5. McIntosh IB, Reed JM, Power KG. The impact of travel acquired illness on the world traveler and family doctor and the need for pre-travel health education. Scott Med J 1994;39(2):40–4.
6. Serafin A. Developing and understanding between people: the key to global health. Travel Med Infect Dis 2010;8:180–3.
7. Gautret P, Schlagenhauf P, Gaudart J, et al. Multicenter EuroTravNet/Geosentinal study of travel-related infectious diseases in Europe. Emerg Infect Dis 2009; 15(11):1783–90.
8. Gautret P, Freedman DO. Travel medicine, a specialty on the move [editorial]. Clin Microbiol Infect 2010;16:201–2.
9. Schlagenhauf P, Santos-O'Connor F, Parola P. The practice of travel medicine in Europe. Clin Microbiol Infect 2010;16:203–8.
10. Hill DR, Bia FJ. Coming of age of travel medicine and tropical diseases: a need for continued advocacy and mentorship. Infect Dis Clin North Am 2005;19:xv–xxi.
11. Jong EC, McMullen R. Travel medicine problems encountered in emergency departments. Emerg Med Clin North Am 1997;15:261–81.
12. Durham MJ, Goad JA, Neinstein LS, et al. A comparison of pharmacist travel-health specialists' versus primary care providers' recommendations for travel-related medications, vaccinations, and patient compliance in a college health setting. J Travel Med 2011;18:20–5.
13. Hatz C, Krause E, Grundmann H. Travel advice: a study among Swiss and German general practitioners. Trop Med Int Health 1997;2(1):6–12.
14. Sofarelli TA, Ricks JH, Anand R, et al. Standardized training in nurse model travel clinics. J Travel Med 2011;18:39–43.
15. Freedman DO, Weld LH, Kozarsky P, et al. Spectrum of disease and relation to place of exposure among ill returned travelers. N Engl J Med 2006;354:119–30.
16. Kotton CN, Hibberd PL, the AST Infectious Diseases Community of Practice. Travel medicine and the solid organ transplant patient. Am J Transplant 2009;9(4):S273–81.
17. Bhadelia N, Klotman M, Caplivski D. The HIV-positive traveler. Am J Med 2007; 120(7):574–80.
18. Han P, Balaban V, Marano C. Travel characteristics and risk-taking attitudes in youths traveling to nonindustrialized countries. J Travel Med 2010;17:316–21.
19. Gautret P, Wilder-Smith A. Vaccination against tetanus, diphtheria, pertussis and poliomyelitis in adult travelers. Travel Med Infect Dis 2010;8:155–60.

20. Centers for Disease Control and Prevention (CDC). Recommended adult immunization schedule—United States, 2011. MMWR Morb Mortal Wkly Rep 2011;60(4):1–4.
21. Ryan ET, Kain KC. Health advice and immunization for travelers. N Engl J Med 2000;342:1716–25.
22. Leder K, Black J, Obrien D, et al. Malaria in travelers: a review of the GeoSentinel surveillance network. Clin Infect Dis 2004;39:1104–12.
23. Leder K, Tong S, Weld L. Illness in travelers visiting friends and relatives: a review of the geographic risk. Clin Infect Dis 2006;43:1185–93.
24. Pavli A, Maltezou HC. Malaria and travelers visiting friends and relatives. Travel Med Infect Dis 2010;8:161–8.
25. Behrens RH, Stauffer WM, Barnett ED, et al. Travel case scenarios as a demonstration of risk assessment of VFR travelers: introduction to criteria and evidence-based definition and framework. J Travel Med 2010;17(3):153–6.
26. Crompton PD, Pierce SK, Miller LH. Advances and challenges in malaria vaccine development. J Clin Invest 2010;120(12):4168–78.
27. Greenwood B. Immunologic correlates of protection for the RTS, S candidate malaria vaccine. Lancet 2011;11:75–6.
28. Good MF. Our impasse in developing a malaria vaccine. Cell Mol Life Sci 2011; 68:1105–13.
29. Doolan DL. Plasmodium immunomics. Int J Parasitol 2010;41:3–20.
30. Aide P, Aponte JJ, Renom M, et al. Safety, immunogenicity and duration of protection of the RTS, S/AS02D malaria vaccine: one year follow-up of a randomized controlled Phase I/IIb trial. PLoS One 2010;5(11):e138.
31. Alonso PL, Sacarlal J, Aponte JJ, et al. Efficacy of the RTS, S/AS02A vaccine against Plasmodium falciparum infection and disease in young African children: randomized controlled trial. Lancet 2004;364:1411–20.
32. Parekh FK, Moorthy VS. Plasmodium vivax vaccine research: insights from Colombian studies. Am J Trop Med Hyg 2011;84(Suppl 2):1–3.
33. Thomas SJ. The necessity and quandaries of dengue vaccine development. J Infect Dis 2011;203:299–303.
34. Gibbons RV. Dengue conundrums. Int J Antimicrob Agents 2010;36S:S36–9.
35. Whitehorn J, Farrar J. Dengue. Br Med Bull 2010;95:161–73.
36. Trent D, Shin J, Hombach J, et al. WHO Working Group on technical specifications for manufacture and evaluation of dengue vaccines, Geneva, Switzerland. Vaccine 2010;28:8246–55.
37. Murrell S, Wu SC, Butler M. Review of dengue virus and the development of a vaccine. Biotechnol Adv 2011;29:239–47.
38. Ross TM. Dengue virus. Clin Lab Med 2010;30:149–60.
39. Dupont HL. Therapy for and prevention of traveller's diarrhea. Clin Infect Dis 2007;45(S1):S78–84.
40. Dupont HL. New insights and directions in traveler's diarrhea. Gastroenterol Clin North Am 2006;35(2):337–53.
41. Schagenhauf P, Chen LH, Wilson ME, et al. Sex and gender differences in travel-associated disease. Clin Infect Dis 2010;50(6):826–32.
42. Stermer E, Lubezky A, Potasman I, et al. Is traveler's diarrhea a significant risk factor for the development of irritable bowel syndrome? A prospective study. Clin Infect Dis 2006;43:898–901.
43. Connor BA. Sequellae of traveler's diarrhea: focus on postinfectious irritable bowel syndrome. Clin Infect Dis 2005;41(Suppl 8):S577–86.
44. Shlim DR. Looking for evidence that personal hygiene precautions prevent traveller's diarrhea. Clin Infect Dis 2005;41(8):S531–5.

45. Wagner A, Wiedermann U. Traveler's diarrhea—pros and cons of different prophylactic measures. Wien Klin Wochenschr 2009;121(Suppl 3):13–8.
46. Connor BA, Blatter MM, Beran J, et al. Rapid and sustained immune response against hepatitis A and B achieved with combined vaccine using an accelerated administration schedule. J Travel Med 2007;14:9–15.
47. Lyons A, Kanesa-thasan N, Kuschner RA, et al. A phase 2 study of a purified, inactivated virus vaccine to prevent Japanese encephalitis. Vaccine 2007;2: 3445–53.
48. Tauber E, Kollaritsch H, Korinek M, et al. Safety and immunogenicity of a Vero-cell-derived, inactivated Japanese encephalitis vaccine: a non-inferiority, phase III, randomized controlled trial. Lancet 2007;370:1847–53.
49. Marfin AA, Eidex RS, Kozarsky PE. Yellow fever and Japanese Encephalitis vaccines: indications and complications. Infect Dis Clin North Am 2005;19: 151–68.

Passive Immunization

Christopher P. Raab, MD[a,b,c,*]

KEYWORDS

- Immunization • Hepatitis B • Botulism • Tetanus • Rabies
- Cytomegalovirus • Respiratory syncytial virus

The process known as passive immunization employs preformed antibodies provided to an individual that can prevent or treat infectious diseases. Naturally, this occurs with the transfer of antibody from mother to fetus. Nearly 100 years ago, the first attempts at artificial passive immunization were attempted using antibodies present in animal sera. While these sera were able to attack the offending microbe, they were poorly tolerated in people, especially with repeated use, as they themselves had antibodies produced against them, causing potentially serious reactions.

Human immune globulin became available shortly after World War I. At that time it required intramuscular (IM) administration, as intravenous (IV) administration caused severe adverse reactions. In 1981, IV immunoglobulin (IVIG) was approved by the US Food and Drug Administration (FDA) for immunodeficiency. There are several situations in which passive immunization can be used: for persons with congenital or acquired immunodeficiency, prophylactic administration when there is a likelihood of exposure to a particular infection, or treatment of a disease state already acquired by the individual. The specific products available for passive immunization include;

IVIG
Specific immune globulins for IM use
Specific immune globulins for IV administration.

Passive immunization is limited by short duration (typically weeks to months), variable response, and adverse reactions. This article will focus on specific immunoglobulins

The author has nothing to disclose.

[a] Thomas Jefferson University, 1020 Walnut Street, Philadelphia, PA 19107, USA
[b] Division of Diagnostic Referral, Nemours/A.I. duPont Hospital for Children, 1600 Rockland Road, Wilmington, DE 19803, USA
[c] Division of Solid Organ Transplant, Nemours/A.I. duPont Hospital for Children, 1600 Rockland Road, Wilmington, DE 19803, USA
* Division of Diagnostic Referral, Nemours/A.I. duPont Hospital for Children, 1600 Rockland Road, Wilmington, DE 19803.
E-mail address: craab@nemours.org

Prim Care Clin Office Pract 38 (2011) 681–691
doi:10.1016/j.pop.2011.07.006 primarycare.theclinics.com
0095-4543/11/$ – see front matter

in the prevention or treatment of infectious diseases, as these are the most likely scenarios one might encounter in primary care practice. These include hepatitis B, varicella, cytomegalovirus, botulism, rabies, tetanus, as well as the monoclonal antibody prophylaxis of respiratory syncytial virus.

IVIG

Pooled immune globulin is used for many purposes in today's medical world. Indications for IVIG include but are not limited to the treatment of antibody deficiency, immune thrombocytopenic purpura, Kawasaki disease, certain seizure disorders, and many inflammatory and immunoregulatory diseases. This article will concentrate on immune globulins specifically for infectious diseases.

SPECIFIC IMMUNE GLOBULINS

High-titer immune globulin preparations are identical to regular formulations of immune globulin except they are derived from patients who are hyperimmunized or convalescing from a specific infection, or from donors who happen to have very high titers to a specific antigen.

HEPATITIS B IMMUNOGLOBULIN

Hepatitis B is a member of the DNA-containing hepadnaviruses and is typically transmitted through blood or bodily fluids. Its presence is a global health problem. Perinatal transmission usually occurs during contact with bodily fluids during delivery and is very efficient. Infection rates in infants born to hepatitis B-infected mothers can be as high as 90%.[1] In the United States, the current incidence (2007) of acute hepatitis B is about 1.5 cases per 100,000 population. This is approximately an 81% decrease since 1990. This is most likely due to active hepatitis B vaccination. Hepatitis B immunoglobulin (HBIG) provides passive protection if given shortly before or soon after exposure to hepatitis B virus. Passive protection is immediate, but temporary, lasting only 3 to 6 months.[2]

Passive immunization in hepatitis B is used in 3 circumstances: prevention of perinatal transmission, exposure in vaccine nonresponders, and prevention of hepatitis B recurrence in liver transplant patients. Current guidelines suggest that pregnant women be screened for hepatitis B at the first prenatal visit, as well as upon admission to hospital for delivery if the woman has an unknown hepatitis surface antigen (HepBsAg) status or risk factors for acquiring hepatitis B.[3]

Newborns are most likely to be exposed to hepatitis B during delivery via exposure to maternal blood. Infants born to mothers who are positive for HepBsAg should receive both hepatitis B vaccine and HBIG within 12 hours of birth. These infants also require completion of the vaccine series by 6 months of age. For mothers whose hepatitis B status is unknown, the vaccine should be given within 12 hours of birth, and the mother's HepBsAg status should be checked. If positive, HBIG should be given. A Cochrane review in 2006 showed that hepatitis vaccination combined with HBIG was superior to hepatitis B vaccine alone.[4] This study also showed that either immunoglobulin administration or vaccination was better than no prophylaxis.[4]

Algorithm for assessment of infant based on maternal HepBsAg status

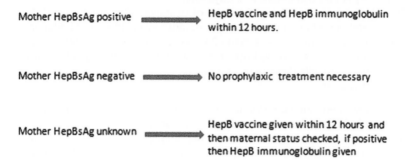

Mother HepBsAg positive →	HepB vaccine and HepB immunoglobulin within 12 hours.
Mother HepBsAg negative →	No prophylaxic treatment necessary
Mother HepBsAg unknown →	HepB vaccine given within 12 hours and then maternal status checked, if positive then HepB immunoglobulin given

Individuals who have been exposed and are unvaccinated or are nonresponders to vaccination should receive hepatitis B vaccine as soon as possible and within 12 hours of the exposure. If the exposure source is known to be HepBsAg positive, HBIG should be administered at the time of vaccination but at a different site than the vaccine. If a person has been exposed but received and responded to the vaccine, no prophylaxis is necessary.

For liver transplant patients who are hepatitis B positive, post-transplant HBIG plus antiviral is the gold standard. This combination therapy has been shown to reduce recurrence rates down to 5% at 5 years after transplant.[5] Some recent studies have looked at withdrawal of HBIG after a finite period of time (typically 1–2 years). While some short-term studies look promising,[6,7] several other studies have shown that switching to lamivudine monotherapy may not provide as much protection as is needed.[8] Improved nucleos(t)ide analogs may make earlier cessation of HBIG in post-liver transplant patients more feasible.[9]

VARICELLA

As a very contagious viral infection, primary varicella has postexposure incidence rates as high as 90% in the nonimmune.[10] Evidence of immunity can be from documentation of immunization, diagnosis of prior disease, or laboratory evidence of antibody. Passive immunization for varicella has a long history dating back to the 1940s using IM immune globulin (IMIG).[11] Eventually, varicella zoster immune globulin (VZIG) was found to be effective in preventing varicella infection in immunocompromised children who had been exposed to varicella.[12] Unfortunately, while VZIG demonstrated it was more effective than prior studies on untreated patients, still 60% of treated patients developed disease. VZIG became unavailable in 2006. Currently VariZig (Cangene Corporation, Winnipeg, Canada) is the sole high-titer varicella immune globulin product. If needed, it can be obtained through an expanded access protocol through its US supplier. Should VariZig be unavailable, IVIG can be used as a substitute but will likely have a lower titer than VariZig.

Patients without varicella immunity who are at high risk for severe disease and have been exposed to varicella are eligible to receive VariZig under the expanded access protocol. The patient groups recommended by the Advisory Committee on Immunization Practices (ACIP) to receive VariZIG include the following[13]

Immunocompromised patients
Neonates whose mothers have signs and symptoms of varicella around the time of delivery (ie, 5 days before to 2 days after)
Premature infants born at $\geq$28 weeks of gestation who are exposed during the neonatal period and whose mothers do not have evidence of immunity
Premature infants born at less than <28 weeks of gestation or who weigh $\leq$1000 g at birth and were exposed during the neonatal period, regardless of maternal history of varicella disease or vaccination
Pregnant women.

Nonimmune pregnant women who are exposed to varicella should be treated with VariZIG within 96 hours of exposure. This can prevent the illness or lessen its severity. If VariZIG is not available, providers can use immune globulin. It is not yet known whether giving varicella zoster immune globulin to a pregnant woman helps to protect the fetus from infection.[14]

The decision for or against immunoprophylaxis depends upon the patient's immune composition and type of exposure. Most immunocompromised patients with prior varicella infection should be considered immune, but those patients who have received a bone marrow transplant should be considered susceptible. Adults and children who are immunocompromised and not vaccinated should be considered susceptible. In patients who are unvaccinated and immunocompromised, varicella titers may be falsely elevated due to possible prior receipt of blood products. As for the type of exposure, concerning contacts include household exposures, face-to-face contact, or contact with a varicella vaccine recipient with a varicella rash.

There are several subsets of patients who are candidates for varicella immune globulin. Newborn infants born to mothers who develop skin findings within 5 days before delivery or 2 days after delivery should receive immune globulin. This time frame does not allow for transfer of maternal antibody. Likewise, all exposed premature infants less than 28 weeks gestation should also receive immune globulin. All susceptible pregnant women are also candidates for immune globulin due to their risk of severe disease.[10] These situations are in addition to the use of varicella immune globulin in immunocompromised patients without a history of varicella disease and without evidence of immunization.

VariZig should be administered within 96 hours of exposure at a dose of 125 U/10 kg intramuscularly. The minimum dose is 125 U and maximum is 625 U. Should VariZig not be available within the appropriate time frame, IVIG at a dose of 400 mg/kg would be an acceptable alternative.

RABIES

Rabies virus (genus *Lyssavirus* family *Rhabdoviridae*) causes a severe progressive encephalomyelitis, which, if untreated, is usually fatal. It is caused by transmission of the virus through saliva in a bite wound from an affected animal. Rabies was one of the earliest diseases studied in terms of passive immunization. This virus made a relatively easy target for studies, as the exposure's time and site are known. Rabies serum was experimented with as early as the 1880s.[15,16] In 1950, the World Health Organization (WHO) recommended studies be performed, and these initial studies demonstrated superiority of a 2-dose antirabies serum over vaccine alone or 1-dose regimen.[17]

Since 1971, human rabies immune globulin (RIG) has been available and is preferred over equine antiserum due to fewer side effects. Current WHO guidelines for postexposure prophylaxis of rabies consist of 3 important steps[18]:

1. Thorough washing of wound with soap solution followed by povidone–iodine
2. Active immunization
3. Passive immunization with rabies antibody.

RIG is recommended in nonimmunized patients for mammalian bites where rabies cannot be ruled out. It is also used for individuals who have exposure to animals suspected of being rabid. In these situations, the recommended dose is 20 IU/kg. This dose should be infiltrated around the wound site to assist in neutralizing the virus.[19] If there are multiple wounds, the RIG should be diluted two- to threefold in saline to acquire enough for wound infiltration.[20] If RIG is not immediately available, the vaccine should be given, and, when available, RIG should be given within the next 7 days.[21]

TETANUS

Tetanus is caused by a neurotoxin released by *Clostridium tetani,* which manifests as severe muscular spasms and trismus. This neurotoxin is released within wounds, and symptoms occur over the next several days.

Tetanus-specific immune globulin is the oldest known specific globulin. In 1890, Behring and Kitasato introduced equine tetanus antitoxin for the treatment of tetanus.[21] Due to the side effects of the equine antitoxin, human tetanus immune globulin (TIG) was developed in the 1960s. It acts by neutralizing toxin before it is transported systemically to the nervous system, and by neutralizing toxin locally to prevent its systemic absorption. Thus, antitoxin can be given locally, at the site of production of toxin (eg, at the site of a wound), intravenously (in severe cases), or intramuscularly (in less severe cases).

Prophylactically, if a nonimmunized person sustains a serious injury or a bite, 250 U to 500 U of TIG should be given intramuscularly as soon as possible.[22] IVIG also can be used if TIG is not available at a dose of 400 mg/kg. If TIG and IVIG are unavailable, 3000 U to 5000 U of tetanus antitoxin (equine) can be administered (after screening and testing for serum sensitivity).[18]

TIG is currently recommended for those who have been exposed to deep wounds and for treatment after exposure. In the event of a dirty wound, the first step of care is cleaning and debriding, as dirty wounds with devascularized tissue are prime targets of *C tetani*. Typically penicillin G is also given, as *C tetani* is typically sensitive. At least 500 U of TIG is recommended, but doses as high as 3000 U to 6000 U have been used.[21] Part of the TIG should be infiltrated near the wound, and the remainder should be given as a single dose intramuscularly. Intrathecal TIG has been tried, but results are conflicting.[23,24] IVIG also contains antibodies to tetanus and can be given if TIG is not available. If TIG and IVIG are unavailable, as is the case in many developing countries, equine tetanus antitoxin can be given in a single dose of 100,000 U, with 50,000 U given intramuscularly and 50,000 intravenously (after appropriate testing for sensitivity). The patient should then undergo primary active immunization.

CYTOMEGALOVIRUS

Cytomegalovirus (CMV) is a herpes virus that is a very common source of infection within the general population. While in immunocompetent patients, CMV typically presents with a wide range of symptoms, it is typically a self-limiting viral syndrome.

In both bone marrow and solid organ transplantation patients, CMV disease can be devastating. Initial studies in the 1980s demonstrated a hyperimmune CMV immune globulin product was efficacious in renal transplants patients.[25] This efficacy was also later demonstrated in the liver,[26] heart,[27] and lung transplant patients.[28] While initially given to most post-transplant patients, eventually it was shown to be of little benefit to bone marrow transplant patients where both the donor and recipient were CMV negative.[29] In most programs, CMV immune globulin is now reserved for patients at high risk (donor positive and recipient negative, having received antilymphocyte antibodies) or intermediate risk (donor positive and recipient positive, or donor negative and recipient positive).[30] Further studies have demonstrated that using CMV immune globulin in combination with gangciclovir was superior to just gangciclovir alone.[31,32] The use of CMV immune globulin in the treatment of severe disease along with antivirals has been beneficial in many studies.[33,34]

Another potential use for CMV immune globulin is in the prevention/treatment of perinatal CMV infection. Several studies have been performed giving pregnant mothers with primary CMV disease CMV immune globulin, either intraperitoneally, within the amniotic sac or umbilical cord, or intravenously.[35,36] In 1 study only 1 mother of 31 in the study gave birth to a child with CMV infection, versus 7 of 14 in the control group.[31] While not recommended for routine pregnancies, this may offer some benefit in certain situations.

BOTULISM

Botulism is caused by ingestion or absorption of spores from *C botulinum*. There are various types of clinical scenarios, including food poisoning through contaminated canned foods, wound contamination, and infant botulism. In infant botulism and its adult counterpart (adult-type infant botulism), spores are ingested and multiply in the gastrointestinal tract, where paralytic toxin is released.

With the exception of infant botulism, other types are typically treated with equine antitoxin as quickly after exposure as possible given intravenously.

For infant botulism, the treatment of choice is human botulism IVIG. Botulism immune globulin IV (BIG-IV), a human-derived botulinum antitoxin, is safe and effective therapy for infant botulism and should be administered as early as possible.[37] Treatment should not be delayed while awaiting results of confirmatory tests. If there is a suspected case of infant botulism, BIG-IV can be obtained through the California Department of Health Services, Infant Botulism Treatment and Prevention Program.

In a randomized controlled trial of 122 infants with infant botulism, BIG-IV was demonstrated to be superior to placebo with respect to reduced mean duration of hospital stay, reduced mean duration of intensive care, reduced mechanical ventilation, and reduced tube or intravenous feeding. No serious adverse events were associated with BIG-IV therapy. Management of infant botulism is otherwise supportive and includes close monitoring to detect sudden worsening. Antibiotics are not indicated for infants with suspected gastrointestinal botulism because of concern that lysis of intraluminal *C botulinum* could increase the amount of toxin available for absorption.

MONOCLONAL ANTIBODY

Unlike other forms of antibodies, monoclonal antibodies are created to bind to a specific receptor or infective agent. These have been used in many fields including as immunosuppressants, antitumor agents, and antivirals.

RESPIRATORY SYNCYTIAL VIRUS

Palivizumab is a monoclonal antibody designed as a prophylactic agent against respiratory syncytial virus (RSV). The virus is a member of the family *Paramyxoviridae* and the subfamily *Pneumovirinae*. It is an enveloped RNA virus, and 2 strains (subgroups A and B) are recognized, the clinical significance of which is unclear. RSV is a very contagious and serious cause of morbidity in infants and young children. Almost all children will have had an RSV infection by their second birthday. RSV causes respiratory illness in infants and young children, and is the most important cause of bronchiolitis. More than 125,000 hospitalizations due to RSV infection occur annually in the United States. Approximately 2% to 3% of all infants in the first 12 months of life will be hospitalized because of an RSV infection.[38] While primarily associated with infants, RSV can also be a serious illness in immunocompromised and the elderly patients.

In 1996, the FDA approved a preventative treatment for RSV using plasma taken from large numbers of normal, healthy individuals containing a high concentration of protective antibodies against RSV (RSVIG). These antibodies do not prevent RSV infections, but do help protect children against the most serious consequences of the virus. In large multicentered controlled studies, RSVIG was shown to reduce hospitalizations among high-risk infants by as much as 68%.[39,40] It is no longer available, because RSVIG is a pooled blood product that has the potential to interfere with some vaccines as well as potentially transmit infectious agents.

Palivizumab was approved by the FDA in 1998. As a humanized monoclonal antibody against a glycoprotein on the virus, it is estimated to have 50 to 100 times more activity than RSVIG. The IMpact-RSV study was a randomized, double-blind, placebo-controlled trial conducted at 139 centers in the United States, the United Kingdom, and Canada. It studied over 1500 high-risk infants and found a 55% reduction in hospitalization as a result of RSV. Children with prematurity but without BPD had a 78% reduction in RSV hospitalization (8.1% vs 1.8%); children with bronchopulmonary dysplasia (BPD) had a 39% reduction (12.8% vs 7.9%). The treatment group had fewer total RSV hospital days and fewer RSV hospital days with increased oxygen.[41]

The American Academy of Pediatrics (AAP) released its first guidelines on the use of palivizumab in 1998, which have been revised most recently in 2009. Initially neither RSVIG nor paliviimab were recommended for children with cyanotic congenital heart disease.[42] In 2003, a randomized, double-blind, placebo-controlled trial conducted by the Cardiac Synagis Group included 1287 children with cyanotic heart disease demonstrated that palivizumab recipients had a 45% relative reduction in RSV hospitalizations and a 56% reduction in total days of RSV hospitalization.[43] In 2009, the AAP published a policy statement regarding palivizumab eligibility. Eligible patients include:[44]

- Infants and children younger than 24 months of age who receive medical therapy (supplemental oxygen, bronchodilator, diuretic, or chronic corticosteroid therapy) for chronic lung disease (CLD) within 6 months before the start of the RSV season; these infants and young children should receive a maximum of 5 doses
- Infants born before 32 weeks' gestation (31 weeks, 6 days or less) may benefit from RSV prophylaxis, even if they do not have CLD; these infants and young children should receive a maximum of 5 doses
  - Infants born at 28 weeks of gestation or earlier may benefit from prophylaxis during the RSV season, whenever that occurs during the first 12 months of life

Infants born at 29 to 32 weeks of gestation may benefit most from prophylaxis if younger than 6 months of age at the start of the RSV season

Infants born at 32 to less than 35 weeks' gestation (defined as 32 weeks, 0 days through 34 weeks, 6 days); palivizumab prophylaxis should be limited to infants younger than 3 months of age at the start of the RSV season or who are born during the RSV season and who are likely to have an increased risk of exposure to RSV; RSV infection is more likely to occur and more likely to lead to hospitalization for infants in this age group when they attend child care or have a sibling younger than 5 years of age

Immunoprophylaxis may be considered for infants born before 35 weeks of gestation who have either congenital airway abnormalities or a neuromuscular condition that compromises handling of respiratory secretions; infants and young children in this category should receive a maximum of 5 doses of palivizumab during the first year of life

Children who are 24 months of age or younger with hemodynamically significant cyanotic or acyanotic congenital heart disease may benefit from palivizumab prophylaxis; children younger than 24 months of age with congenital heart disease who are most likely to benefit from immunoprophylaxis include

Infants who are receiving medication to control congestive heart failure

Infants with moderate to severe pulmonary hypertension

Infants with cyanotic heart disease.

A newer monoclonal antibody, motavizumab, has been developed for RSV prophylaxis. Motaviumab possess 18-fold RSV-neutralizing activity, although a recent study demonstrated noninferiority as compared with palivimumab; it did not demonstrate superiority in regards to RSV hospitalizations.[45] It is currently pending FDA approval.

SUMMARY

The use of passive immunization through immunoglobulins is an effective and safe method of dealing with specific infectious diseases. While IVIG can be an effective safety net for postexposure infections, hyperimmune preparations are often more effective, but also more costly. In the future, one can look to monoclonal antibodies to directly and specifically attack microbes of bacterial and viral origins.

REFERENCES

1. Stevens CE, Beasley RP, Tsui J, et al. Vertical transmission of hepatitis B antigen in Taiwan. N Engl J Med 1975;292:771.
2. Previsani N, Lavanchy D, Zuckerman AJ, et al. Viral hepatitis. In: Mushawar IK, editor, Perspectives in medical virology. Amsterdam: Elsevier; 2003. p. 31–98.
3. Mast E, Margolis H, Fiore A, et al. A comprehensive immunization strategy to eliminate transmission of hepatitis B virus infection in the United States, recommendations of the Advisory Committee on Immunization Practices (ACIP) part 1: immunization of infants, children, and adolescents. MMWR Recomm Rep 2005;54(RR16):1–23.
4. Lee C, Gong Y, Brok J, et al. Hepatitis B immunisation for newborn infants of hepatitis B surface antigen-positive mothers. Cochrane Database Syst Rev 2006;2:CD004790.
5. Markowitz JS, Martin P, Conrad AJ, et al. Prophylaxis against hepatitis B recurrence following liver transplantation using combination of lamivudine and hepatitis B immune globulin. Hepatology 1998;28:585–9.

6. Wong SN, Chu CJ, Wai CT, et al. Low-risk of hepatitis B virus recurrence after withdrawal of long-term hepatitis immunoglobulin in patients receiving maintenance nucleos(t)ide analogue therapy. Liver Transpl 2007;13:374–81.
7. Buti M, Mas A, Prieto M, et al. A randomized study comparing lamivudine monotherapy after a short course of hepatitis immunoglobulin (HBIg) and lamivudine with long-term lamivudine plus HBIg in the prevention of hepatitis B virus recurrence after liver transplantation. J Hepatol 2003;38:811–7.
8. Buti M, Mas A, Prieto M, et al. Adherence to lamivudine after an early withdrawal of hepatitis immunoglobulin plays an important role in the long-term prevention of hepatitis B virus recurrence. Transplantation 2007;84:650–4.
9. Patterson SJ, Angus PW. Postliver transplant hepatitis B prophylaxis: the role of oral nucleos(t)ide analogues. Curr Opin Organ Transplant 2009;14: 225–30.
10. Marin M, Guris D, Chaves SS, et al. Prevention of varicella: recommendations of the Advisory Committee on Immunization Practices (ACIP). MMWR Recomm Rep 2007;56(RR04):1–40.
11. Funkhouser WL. The use of gamma globulin antibodies to control chickenpox in a convalescent hospital for children. J Pediatr 1948;32:257–9.
12. Zaia JA, Levin MJ, Preblud SR, et al. Evaluation of varicella-zoster immune globulin: protection of immunosuppressed children after household exposure to varicella. J Infect Dis 1983;147:737.
13. Centers for Disease Control. A new product (VariZIG) for postexposure prophylaxis of varicella available under an investigational new drug application expanded access protocol. MMWR Morb Mortal Wkly Rep 2006;55: 209–10.
14. American Academy of Pediatrics. In: Pickering LK, Baker CJ, Long SS, et al, editors. Red Book: 2006 Report of the Committee on Infectious Diseases. 27th editon. Elk Grove Village (IL): American Academy of Pediatrics; 2006.
15. Babes V, Lepp M. Recherches sur la vaccination antirabique. Ann Inst Pasteur 1889;3:385–90 [in French].
16. Stiehm E, Keller M. Rabies and rabies immune globulin. In: Feigin RD, editor. Feigin and Cherry's textbook of pediatric infectious disease. 6th edition. Philadelphia: Saunders; 2009. p. 3430–1.
17. Baltazard M, Bahmanyar M. Essai pratique du serum antirabique chez les mordus par loups enfantes. Bull World Health Organ 1955;13:747–72 [in French].
18. World Health Organization. Wkly Epidemiol Rec 2010;85:309–20.
19. American Academy of Pediatrics. Rabies. In: Pickering LK, editor. Red Book: 2006 Report of the Committee on Infectious Diseases. 27th editon. Elk Grove Village (IL): American Academy of Pediatrics; 2006. p. 552–9.
20. World Health Organization. WHO recommendations on rabies postexposure treatment and the correct technique, part 1. Guide for rabies postexposure treatment. Geneva (Switzerland): World Health Organization; 1997.
21. Patel JC, Mehta BC, Nanavati BH, et al. Role of serum therapy in tetanus. Lancet 1963;1:740–3.
22. American Academy of Pediatrics. Tetanus (Lockjaw). In: Pickering LK, editor. Red Book: 2006 Report of the Committee on Infectious Diseases. 27th editon. Elk Grove Village (IL): American Academy of Pediatrics; 2006. p. 648–53.
23. Begue RE, Lindo-Soriano I. Failure of intrathecal tetanus antitoxin in the treatment of tetanus neonatorum. J Infect Dis 1991;164:619–20.
24. Gupta PS, Kapoor R, Goyal S, et al. Intrathecal human tetanus immunoglobulin in early tetanus. Lancet 1980;2:439–40.

25. Snydman DR, Werner BG, Heinze-Lacey B, et al. Use of cytomegalovirus immune globulin to prevent cytomegalovirus disease in renal-transplant recipients. N Engl J Med 1987;317:1049–54.
26. Falagas ME, Snydman DR, Ruthazer R, et al. Cytomegalovirus immune globulin (CMVIG) prophylaxis is associated with increased survival after orthotopic liver transplantation. Clin Transplant 1997;11:432–7.
27. Weill D. Role of cytomegalovirus in cardiac allograft vasculopathy. Transpl Infect Dis 2001;3:44–8.
28. Weill D, Lock BJ, Wewers DL, et al. Combination prophylaxis with ganciclovir and cytomegalovirus (CMV) immune globulin after lung transplantation: effective CMV prevention following daclizumab induction. Am J Transplant 2003;3:492–6.
29. Ruutu T, Ljungman P, Brinch L, et al. No prevention of cytomegalovirus infection by anti-cytomegalovirus hyperimmune globulin in seronegative bone marrow transplant recipients. Bone Marrow Transplant 1997;19:233–6.
30. Cytomegalovirus prophylaxis following Solid Organ Transplants Guideteam, Cincinnati Children's Hospital Medical Center: Evidence-based care guideline for CMV Prophylaxis following Solid Organ Transplant. Available at: www.cincinnatichildrens.org/svc/alpha/h/health-policy/ev-based/cmv-transplant.htm. Accessed March 3, 2011. Guideline 17, July 6, 2007. p. 1–16.
31. Snydman DR, Falagas ME, Avery R, et al. Use of combination cytomegalovirus immune globulin plus ganciclovir for prophylaxis in CMV-seronegative liver transplant recipients of a CMV-seropositive donor organ: a multicenter, open-label study. Transplant Proc 2001;33:2571–5.
32. Ruttmann E, Geltner C, Bucher B, et al. Combined CMV prophylaxis improves outcome and reduces the risk for bronchiolitis obliterans syndrome (BOS) after lung transplantation. Transplantation 2006;81:1415–20.
33. Reed EC, Bowden RA, Dandliker PS, et al. Treatment of cytomegalovirus pneumonia with ganciclovir and intravenous cytomegalovirus immunoglobulin in patients with bone marrow transplants. Ann Intern Med 1988;109:783–8.
34. Paar DP, Pollard RB. Immunotherapy of CMV infections. Adv Exp Med Biol 1996; 394:145–51.
35. Nigro G, Adler SP, La Torre R, et al. Passive immunization during pregnancy for congenital cytomegalovirus infection. N Engl J Med 2005;353:1350–62, 422.
36. Negishi H, Yamada H, Hirayama E, et al. Intraperitoneal administration of cytomegalovirus hyperimmunoglobulin to the cytomegalovirus-infected fetus. J Perinatol 1998;18:466–9.
37. American Academy of Pediatrics. Botulism and infant botulism. In: Pickering LK, editor. Red Book: 2006 Report of the Committee on Infectious Diseases. 27th editon. Elk Grove Village (IL): American Academy of Pediatrics; 2006. p. 259.
38. Meissner HC, Bocchini J. *Reducing RSV hospitalizations*, AAP modifies recommendations for use of palivizumab in high-risk infants, young children. AAP News 2009;30(7):1.
39. Reduction of respiratory syncytial virus hospitalization among premature infants and infants with bronchopulmonary dysplasia using respiratory syncytial virus immune globulin prophylaxis. Pediatrics 1997;99:93.
40. Groothius JR, Simoes EA, Levin MJ, et al. Prophylactic administration of respiratory syncytial virus immune globulin to high-risk infants and young children. The Respiratory Syncytial Virus Immune Globulin Study Group. N Engl J Med 1993;329:1524.
41. The IMpact RSV Study Group. Palivizumab, a humanized respiratory syncytial virus monoclonal antibody, reduces hospitalization from respiratory syncytial virus infection in high-risk infants. Pediatrics 1998;102:531–7.

42. American Academy of Pediatrics Committee on Infectious Diseases and Committee of Fetus and Newborn. Prevention of respiratory syncytial virus infections: indications for the use of palivizumab and update on the use of RSV-IVIG. Pediatrics 1998;102(5):1211–6.
43. Feltes TF, Cabalka AK, Meissner HC, et al. Palivizumab prophylaxis reduces hospitalization due to respiratory syncytial virus in young children with hemodynamically significant congenital heart disease. J Pediatr 2003;143:532.
44. American Academy of Pediatrics Committee on Infectious Diseases. Policy statement—modified recommendations for use of palivizumab for the prevention of respiratory syncytial virus infections. Pediatrics 2009;124:1684–701.
45. Carbonell-Estrany X, Simões EA, Dagan R, et al. Motavizumab for prophylaxis of respiratory syncytial virus in high-risk children: a noninferiority trial. Pediatrics 2010;125:e35–51.

The Course and Management of the 2009 H1N1 Pandemic Influenza

Sanford R. Kimmel, MD

KEYWORDS

- Pandemic H1N1 influenza • Epidemiology • Diagnosis
- Immunization

PAST EPISODES OF PANDEMIC INFLUENZA

The recent pandemic influenza of 2009 caused major concern among public health authorities and the general public. Frequent reminders were made to the 3 worldwide (pandemic) outbreaks of the twentieth century: the "Spanish" flu of 1918, the "Asian" flu of 1957, and the "Hong Kong" flu of 1968.[1] The "Spanish" influenza epidemic of 1918 to 1919 is the most infamous, and is estimated at infecting 500 million persons and killing 50 to 100 million people worldwide.[2] All subsequent influenza A pandemics are believed to have been caused by the descendants of the 1918 virus, which still persist in pigs.[2] The origin of the 1918 avian-like influenza virus remains unknown, but humans and pigs had no immunity to it.[2] Although most patients experienced typical influenza symptoms, the lack of antibiotics to combat bacterial superinfections and the chaos of World War I played a role in the high mortality rate.

THE SPREAD OF 2009 INFLUENZA A (H1N1) PANDEMIC

In March 2009, a respiratory illness caused by swine-origin influenza A (H1N1) virus (S-OIV) was identified in Mexico. By May 29, 2009, Mexico reported more than 4900 confirmed cases and 85 deaths due to S-OIV.[3] The first reported S-OIV cases in the United States occurred in California on March 28 and 30, 2009. From April 15 through May 5, 2009, 642 confirmed cases of S-OIV influenza were reported in 41 states.[4] The most common symptoms in this series were fever (94%), cough (92%), sore throat (66%), diarrhea (25%) and vomiting (25%).[4] Following reports from countries such as New Zealand, Spain, and the United Kingdom, the pandemic alert

Disclosure: Dr Kimmel owns 100 shares of GlaxoSmithKline.

Department of Family Medicine, University of Toledo College of Medicine, Mail Stop 1179, 3000 Arlington Avenue, Toledo, OH 43614, USA
E-mail address: Sanford.Kimmel@utoledo.edu

Prim Care Clin Office Pract 38 (2011) 693–701
doi:10.1016/j.pop.2011.07.007 primarycare.theclinics.com

phases were raised to level 5 (**Table 1**) by April 29.[5] The United States and Canada subsequently reported 745 and 201 confirmed cases, respectively, with sporadic reports from other countries.[5] On June 11, 2009, the World Health Organization (WHO) raised the pandemic alert to phase 6, officially recognizing that influenza A (H1N1) was characterized by sustained human-to-human transmission with outbreaks in at least one country in two or more WHO regions.[6]

In all countries most reported cases of pandemic influenza occurred in children, adolescents, and young adults, who also comprised a higher percentage of hospitalized cases. Comorbidities such as asthma, pregnancy, and diabetes increased the severity of disease and rates of hospitalization.[6] A single-center study also observed that obesity seemed to be a risk factor for hospitalization and influenza-related complications, but was too small to demonstrate significance,[7] Children admitted to the Toronto Hospital for Sick Children for H1N1 influenza during 2009 were significantly older than those with seasonal influenza (median age 6.4 years vs 3.3 years) and more likely to have asthma (22.2% vs 6%).[8] Seventeen of 58 children (29%) in this study also had radiographic evidence of pneumonia.[8] In a study of all Australian and New Zealand intensive care units (ICUs), a higher risk of ICU admission was found in pregnant women, adults with a body mass index greater than 35 kg/m^2, and indigenous Australian and New Zealand populations with confirmed H1N1 infection.[9]

In the United States, the Centers for Disease Control and Prevention (CDC) estimated that 43 to 89 million H1N1 infections occurred from April 2009 through April 2010, with more than an estimated 270,000 hospitalizations and 12,000 deaths.[10] A Wisconsin study of more than half a million cases found that H1N1-infected individuals were younger than those infected with H3N2 influenza, but with no increased risk of serious complications.[10] Unlike typical seasonal influenza, adults older than 60 years have been less susceptible to H1N1, possibly because of exposure to antigenically similar viruses. A CDC study found that 39 of 115 persons (34%) born before 1950 had titers of 80 against 2009 H1N1 influenza whereas only 4 of 107 (4%) persons

Table 1
World Health Organization influenza pandemic phases

Interpandemic Period	
Phase 1	No new influenza virus subtypes detected in humans. An influenza virus subtype that has caused human infection may be present in animals. If present in animals, the risk of human disease is considered to be low
Phase 2	No new influenza virus subtypes detected in humans. A circulating animal influenza virus subtype poses a substantial risk of human disease
Pandemic Alert Period	
Phase 3	Human infection(s) with a new influenza virus subtype, but no human-to-human spread, or at most rare instances of spread to a close contact
Phase 4	Small cluster(s) of disease with limited human-to-human transmission but highly localized spread suggesting virus is not well adapted to humans
Phase 5	Larger cluster(s) but human-to-human spread still localized, suggesting that the virus is becoming increasingly better adapted to humans, but may not yet be fully transmissible (substantial pandemic risk)
Pandemic Period	
Phase 6	Pandemic phase: increased and sustained transmission in the general population
Postpandemic Period	
Phase 1	Return to Interpandemic period (Phase 1)

born after 1980 had preexisting cross-reactive titers of 40 or more.[11] A Canadian study found that persons born before 1957 had a lower risk of infection (adjusted odds ratio of 0.15) whereas those born between 1957 and 1975 had an intermediate risk of infection (adjusted odds ratio 0.42) compared with those 33 years old or younger.[12] Younger persons were considered more susceptible to H1N1with estimates of infection in Pittsburgh at 21% of all persons and 45% of those between the ages of 10 and 19 years.[13] The crystal structure of the soluble hemagglutinin 09H1 of the 2009 S-OIV is very similar to the 1918 pandemic influenza 18H1 and distinct from that of the seasonal flu viruses.[14] This antigenic similarity at least partially explains why older adults previously exposed to the 1918 virus or similar strains have cross-reactivity and protection to the 2009 H1N1 influenza virus.

RISK FACTORS FOR INFLUENZA A (H1N1) INFECTION

The 2009 H1N1 influenza virus has a person-to-person transmission similar to seasonal influenza, but the contributions of small-droplet versus large-droplet aerosols and fomites are unknown.[15] Most illnesses caused by the 2009 H1N1 virus were acute and self-limited, but 25% to 50% of patients who were hospitalized or died had no reported coexisting medical conditions. In New York City, pregnant women were more than 7 times more likely to be hospitalized and more than 4 times more likely to be admitted to an ICU from 2009 H1N1 influenza than nonpregnant women.[16] In California, 20% of hospitalized pregnant women with 2009 H1N1 infection required intensive care and accounted for 6% of patients who died.[16] Although the median age of hospitalization in this study was 27 years, infants had the highest rates of hospitalization, and persons 50 years and older had the highest rates of mortality once hospitalized.[17] Risk factors or comorbid conditions that contribute to severe or fatal illness with 2009 H1N1 virus infection are given in **Box 1**.[15,17]

CLINICAL PRESENTATION AND DIAGNOSIS OF INFLUENZA A (H1N1) INFECTIONS

The incubation period of influenza A H1N1 is similar to seasonal influenza at 1.5 to 3 days, but may extend up to 7 days.[15] Most persons have fever and cough that may be accompanied by sore throat and rhinorrhea, although some persons do not have fever. Unlike seasonal influenza, approximately 40% of hospitalized children and adults may have vomiting and diarrhea.[18] Progression of disease is signified by dyspnea, tachypnea, chest pain, production of purulent sputum or hemoptysis, and altered mental status. Diffuse viral pneumonitis associated with severe hypoxemia, adult respiratory distress syndrome (ARDS), and shock or renal failure has accounted for the majority of ICU admissions attributable to the 2009 H1N1 influenza virus.[15] Chest radiographs often demonstrate diffuse mixed interstitial and alveolar infiltrates, but lobar and multilobar infiltrates can occur in patients with bacterial infection. Asthma was present in at least 25% of children and adults who were admitted because of H1N1 virus.[18] Laboratory findings may include normal or low-normal leukocyte counts (20%), anemia (37%), and thrombocytopenia (14%).[18] Elevations of serum aminotransferases, lactate dehydrogenase, creatine kinase, and creatinine may occur, especially if there is associated myositis and rhabdomyolysis.[15]

Because of the lack of specificity in its clinical symptoms and signs, diagnosis of influenza A H1N1 depends on maintaining a high level of clinical suspicion, especially in the setting of an outbreak. Reverse-transcriptase–polymerase chain reaction (RT-PCR) is the best method to detect the viral RNA of 2009 H1N1, especially if the sample can be obtained from the lower respiratory tract.[15] One commercial rapid influenza

Box 1
Risk factors/comorbid conditions for 2009 H1N1 influenza infection

Age <5 years old

Age ≥65 years (low infection rate but high mortality)

American Indians/Alaskan Natives

Asthma

Chronic aspirin therapy in children (due to risk of Reye syndrome)

Chronic cardiovascular disease (except hypertension)

Chronic hepatic disease

Chronic obstructive pulmonary disease or other lung disorder

Chronic renal disease

Diabetes or other metabolic disease

Hemoglobinopathy or other hematologic disorder

Immunosuppression

Neurocognitive disorder

Neuromuscular disorder

Morbid obesity (body mass index ≥35 or 40 kg/m^2)

Pregnancy

Seizure disorder

test (QuickVue Influenza A+B; Quidel, San Diego, CA) demonstrated a sensitivity of 51% for S-OIV compared with RT-PCR assay, although its specificity was 99%.[19]

ANTIVIRAL THERAPY FOR INFLUENZA

The 2009 H1N1 influenza A virus is generally susceptible to the neuraminidase inhibitors oseltamivir (Tamiflu; Roche, Basel, Switzerland) and zanamivir (Relenza; GlaxoSmithKline, Brentford, UK). The adamantanes amantadine and rimantadine are not recommended for antiviral treatment or chemoprophylaxis of influenza A because of resistance in circulating influenza A viruses.[20] Neuraminidase inhibitor therapy is important for patients with at-risk conditions (see **Box 1**), including pregnant women. Recommended doses are given in **Table 2**.[20] In general, oseltamivir and zanamivir have been shown to decrease the duration of uncomplicated influenza A and B by about 1 day if given within 48 hours of symptom onset.[20] Neuraminidase inhibitor administration has also been associated with improved survival rates among patients hospitalized with 2009 H1N1 influenza A.[21] As a result, patients requiring hospitalization with illness suspected or confirmed to be due to H1N1 should be treated, even if they present more than 48 hours after illness onset.[20] A retrospective Chinese study of patients with mild pandemic 2009 influenza suggested that oseltamivir reduced the risk of pneumonia found on chest radiography, and that treatment within 2 days of symptom onset could reduce the duration of fever and viral RNA shedding.[22] In this study, pandemic 2009 H1N1 virus was shed from 1 day before the onset of symptoms to up to 8 days afterward, longer than with seasonal influenza virus.[22] If influenza activity is present in the community, antiviral treatment can be considered for

Table 2
Treatment and chemoprophylaxis of H1N1 influenza with antiviral medications

Age or Population Group	Oseltamivir[a]		Zanamivir[b]	
	Treatment[c]	Prophylaxis[d]	Treatment[c]	Prophylaxis[d]
3–11 mo	3 mg/kg twice daily	3 mg/kg once daily	NA	NA
1–6 y	If ≤15 kg, 30 mg twice daily If >15–23 kg, 45 mg twice daily If >23–40 kg, 60 mg twice daily If >40 kg, 75 mg twice daily	If ≤15 kg, 30 mg once daily If >15–23 kg, 45 mg once daily If >23–40 kg, 60 mg once daily If >40 kg, 75 mg once daily	NA	NA for 1–4 y
5–6 y	Dose varies by weight as above	Dose varies by weight as above	NA	10 mg (2 inhalations) once daily
7–9 y			10 mg (2 inhalations) twice daily	10 mg (2 inhalations) once daily
10–12 y	Dose varies by weight as above If >40 kg, give adult dose	Dose varies by weight as above If >40 kg, give adult dose	10 mg (2 inhalations) twice daily	10 mg (2 inhalations) once daily
13–64 y	75 mg twice daily	75 mg once daily	10 mg (2 inhalations) twice daily	10 mg (2 inhalations) once daily
≥65 y	75 mg twice daily	75 mg once daily	10 mg (2 inhalations) twice daily	10 mg (2 inhalations) once daily

Abbreviation: NA, not available.

[a] Oseltamivir (Tamiflu, Roche Pharmaceuticals) is approved for treatment or chemoprophylaxis of persons ≥1 year old. No antiviral medications are approved for treatment or chemoprophylaxis of children <1 year old. An emergency use authorization was issued by the Food and Drug Administration on April 28, 2009 and expired on June 23, 2010. Weight-based dosing is not appropriate for premature infants who might have slower renal clearance.

[b] Zanamivir is approved for treatment of persons ≥7 years old and for chemoprophylaxis of persons ≥5 years old.

[c] Treatment is recommended for 5 days but can be extended for patients who remain severely ill.

[d] Chemoprophylaxis is recommended for 10 days after a household exposure and 7 days after most recent known exposure in other situations.

Data from Centers for Disease Control and Prevention. Antiviral agents for the treatment and chemoprophylaxis of influenza. MMWR Recomm Rep 2011;60:1–25; Tables 1 and 4.

outpatients with uncomplicated, suspected, or confirmed disease if it can be begun within 48 hours of symptom onset.[19]

EFFECTIVENESS OF THE 2009 H1N1 INFLUENZA VACCINE

By November 2009, the 2009 H1N1 virus was reported to have infected people in more than 190 countries and caused more than 4500 deaths.[23] Once it became apparent that 2009 influenza disease might become pandemic, several developed nations decided to sponsor and promote the production of an influenza vaccine against H1N1. This initiative was possible because the complete genetic sequence of the hemagglutinin (HI) of the virus was rapidly characterized.[24] Because of the development of Guillain-Barré syndrome (GBS) that developed in 1 out of 100,000 persons vaccinated during the swine flu scare of 1976, ongoing safety and efficacy studies were conducted. A small study in Costa Rica found that a single 15-μg dose of 2009 H1N1 vaccine with and without adjuvant met licensure criteria of the Center for Biologic Evaluation and Research (CBER) for children aged 9 to 17 years. Children 3 to 8 years old required a 7.5-μg dose to meet immunogenicity criteria.[25] Seroconversion rates were 70% in all age and vaccine groups.[25] A German study using a monovalent H1N1 vaccine with an adjuvant containing 3.25 μg hemagglutinin (Pandemrix) estimated a vaccine efficacy of more than 95% for persons aged 14 to 59 years and more than 80% for persons 60 years or older.[26]

In the United States, the influenza A (H1N1) California/7/2009-like strain was used in the 2009 monovalent H1N1 vaccine and also in the 2010 trivalent seasonal vaccine. Among children aged 6 to 35 months, HI titers of 40 or greater varied from 19% to 92% after one dose. After 2 doses separated by at least 21 days were given, more than 90% of children developed HI titers of 40 or greater.[27] Among children aged 3 to 9 years, HI titers varied from 44% to 93% after one dose of vaccine while more than 90% developed titers of 40 or greater after 2 doses.[27] Two doses of H1N1 vaccine separated by 4 weeks are consequently recommended for children aged 6 months to 8 years receiving influenza vaccine for the first time. If only one dose has been given for the first time during the preceding year, then 2 doses should be given the following year. Among older children and adults, more than 90% developed suitable response rates to the vaccine.[27]

SAFETY OF THE 2009 H1N1 INFLUENZA VACCINE

Safety is a major concern with the production of any vaccine or biologic compound. Because of the previous association of GBS following the use of the 1976 swine flu vaccine, there was particular concern about the development of GBS with the 2009 H1N1 monovalent vaccine. Some patients who were willing to receive the 2009 seasonal influenza vaccine declined to receive the monovalent 2009 influenza vaccine because it was perceived as a "new" vaccine. The US Food and Drug Administration licensed the 2009 monovalent H1N1 vaccine in 2009 as both a live attenuated vaccine and inactivated, split-virus, or subunit vaccine. Neither vaccine contained adjuvant. Safety data were subsequently reviewed from the by the US Vaccine Adverse Event Reporting System (VAERS) and the Vaccine Safety Datalink (VSD) reporting system. No significant differences between H1N1 and seasonal influenza vaccines were noted in the proportion or types of serious adverse events (SAE).[28] Through November 24, 2009 VAERS reported SAE after H1N1 vaccine and seasonal influenza vaccine of 5.4% and 6.1%, respectively. Four cases of GBS were confirmed after H1N1 vaccine and 4 were under investigation.[28] From October 1 through November 21, more than 400,000 doses of H1N1 vaccine were given to the 9.5 million members of the 8 managed care organizations that comprise the VSD. No cases of GBS and only one case of anaphylaxis were reported in vaccinated persons in the VSD system.[28] From October 1, 2009 through May 10, 2010, the CDC's Emerging Infections Program (EIP), covering approximately 45 million persons in 10 states, found 27 cases of GBS in vaccinated persons and 274 in unvaccinated persons, and estimated an attributable risk of 0.8 excess cases of GBS per 1 million vaccinations.[29] These results are comparable with those of studies in some years of seasonal influenza vaccine, and much less than the 10 excess cases per 1 million vaccinations seen during the 1976 swine flu campaign.[29] Persons who have a history of GBS have a greater likelihood of recurrent symptoms. As a consequence, health care providers do not generally vaccinate persons who are not at high risk for influenza complications and who have had GBS within 6 weeks of previous receipt of an influenza vaccine (trivalent or monovalent).[27] For these persons antiviral chemoprophylaxis should be considered.

IMPLEMENTATION AND COVERAGE WITH THE 2009 H1N1 VACCINE

Several issues were encountered with the production and distribution of the monovalent 2009 H1N1 vaccine. Production of the vaccine took longer than anticipated, delaying shipment and distribution into the community until October 2009. Health care providers including public health authorities often did not know when they would receive shipments and how many doses they would contain. Initially many vaccination clinics were held on short notice with long lines of people waiting to be immunized. In some areas, sufficient or even excessive amounts of vaccine were available, leading to a mismatch of supply and demand. Once significant quantities of vaccine became available, a perception that the epidemic was beginning to wane lessened demand for the vaccine. In fact, the WHO declared the end of phase 6 of pandemic influenza on August 10, 2010, stating that the H1N1 virus had run its course.[30]

From August 2009 through May 2010 the CDC estimated that 27% of all persons in the United States. aged 6 months and older were vaccinated with the 2009 H1N1 vaccine compared with 41.2% receiving the seasonal vaccine.[31] Among children 6 months to 17 years old, vaccination coverage was 40.5% for H1N1 versus 43.7% for the seasonal vaccine.[31] Thirty-eight percent of adults aged 18 to 49 years with high-risk conditions received H1N1 versus 28% of those without high-risk conditions who received seasonal influenza vaccine.[32] The CDC estimated that 31.6 million children and 91.6 million adults were given one or more seasonal vaccine doses. An estimated 29.3 million children and 51.5 million adults were administered one or more doses of 2009 H1N1 vaccine.[31] A 10-state study of pregnant women found that 50.7% reported receiving seasonal influenza vaccine versus 46.6% for 2009 H1N1.[32] Almost 25% to 30% of patients reported that their provider did not mention either vaccine, while approximately 45% of patients offered seasonal vaccine were concerned about side effects to them or their baby.[32] Similarly, more than 60% of pregnant women were concerned about the effects of the H1N1 vaccine on them or their baby.[32] However, after demonstrating its safety and efficacy, the 2009 H1N1 vaccine was incorporated as 1 of 3 components in the 2010 seasonal influenza vaccine.[27,33]

SUMMARY

During typical influenza seasons most influenza-associated hospitalizations occur among persons 65 years and older. During the 2009 H1N1 pandemic, younger persons accounted for the majority of hospitalizations, with 280 pediatric deaths associated with laboratory-confirmed H1N1 virus reported from April 26, 2009 through April 16, 2010.[33] Approximately two-thirds of these children had medical conditions placing them at high risk, emphasizing the need to vaccinate these populations. The length of time required to bring the new vaccine to market using existing vaccine production methodologies emphasized the need to expedite this process by using different and faster technologies. The epidemic also demonstrated that vaccine distribution must be more accurately matched to areas of vaccine need. Fortunately, the 2009 influenza H1N1 pandemic was not as devastating as feared. It provided a good test of the nation's current public health capabilities and helped to identify areas where improvement is needed.

REFERENCES

1. Kilbourne ED. Influenza pandemics of the 20th century. Emerg Infect Dis 2006; 12:9–14. Available at: www.cdc.gov/eid. Accessed April 4, 2011.
2. Taubenberger JK, Morens DM. 1918 influenza: the mother of all pandemics. Emerg Infect Dis 2006;12:15–22.
3. Perez-Padilla R, de la Rosa-Zamboni D, Ponce de Leon S, et al. Pneumonia and respiratory failure from swine-origin influenza A (H1N1) in Mexico. N Engl J Med 2009;361:680–9.
4. Novel Swine-Origin Influenza A (H1N1) Virus Investigation Team. Emergence of a novel swine-origin influenza A (H1N1) virus in humans. N Engl J Med 2009; 360:2605–15.
5. EDC Technical Emergency Team. Initial epidemiological findings in the European Union following the declaration of pandemic alert level 5 due to influenza A (H1N1). Euro Surveill 2009;14(18):1–4.
6. New influenza A (H1N1) virus: global epidemiological situation, June 2009. Wkly Epidemiol Rec 2009;84:249–60 [in English, French].
7. Plessa E, Diakakis P, Gardelis J, et al. Clinical features, risk factors, and complications among pediatric patients with pandemic influenza A (H1N1). Clin Pediatr (Phila) 2010;49:777–81.
8. O'Riordan S, Barton M, Yau Y, et al. Risk factors and outcomes among children admitted to hospital with pandemic H1N1 influenza. CMAJ 2010;182:39–44.
9. The ANZIC Influenza Investigators. Critical care services and 2009 H1N1 influenza in Australia and New Zealand. N Engl J Med 2009;361:1925–34.
10. Belongia EA, Irving SA, Waring SC, et al. Clinical characteristics and 30-day outcomes for influenza A 2009 (H1N1), 2008-2009 (H1N1), and 2007-2008 (H3N2) infections. JAMA 2010;304(10):1091–8.
11. Hancock K, Veguilla V, Lu X, et al. Cross-reactive antibody responses to the 2009 pandemic H1N1 influenza virus. N Engl J Med 2009;361:1945–52.
12. Fishman DN, Savage R, Gubbay J, et al. Older age and reduced likelihood of 2009 H1N1 virus infection. N Engl J Med 2009;361:2000–1.
13. Ross T, Zimmer S, Burke D, et al. Seroprevalence following the second wave of pandemic 2009 H1N1 influenza. PLoS Curr Influenza 2010; RRN1148.
14. Zhang W, Qi J, Shi Y, et al. Crystal structure of the swine-origin (H1N1)-2009 influenza A virus hemagglutinin (HA) reveals similar antigenicity to that of the 1918 pandemic virus. Protein Cell 2010;1(5):459–67.
15. Bautista E, Chotpitayasunondh T, Gao Z, et al. Clinical aspects of pandemic (H1N1) 2009 influenza. Clinical aspects of pandemic 2009 influenza A (H1N1) virus infection. N Engl J Med 2010;362:1708–19.
16. Centers for Disease Control & Prevention. 2009 Pandemic influenza A(H1N1) in pregnant women requiring intensive care—New York City, 2009. MMWR Morb Mortal Wkly Rep 2010;59:321–6.

17. Louie JK, Acosta M, Winter K, et al. Factors associated with death or hospitalization due to pandemic 2009 influenza A (H1N1) infection in California. JAMA 2009; 302:1896–902.
18. Jain S, Kamimoto L, Bramley AM, et al. Hospitalized patients with 2009 H1N1 influenza in the United States, April—June 2009. N Engl J Med 2009;361:1935–44.
19. Faix DJ, Sherman SS, Waterman SH. Rapid-test sensitivity for novel swine-origin influenza A (H1N1) virus in humans. N Engl J Med 2009;361:728–9.
20. Centers for Disease Control & Prevention. Antiviral agents for the treatment and chemoprophylaxis of influenza. MMWR Recomm Rep 2011;60:1–25.
21. Dominquez-Cherit G, Lapinsky SE, Macias AE, et al. Critically ill patients with 2009 influenza A(H1N1) in Mexico. JAMA 2009;302:1880–7.
22. Yu H, Liao Q, Yuan Y, et al. Effectiveness of oseltamivir on disease progression and viral RNA shedding in patients with mild pandemic 2009 influenza A H1N1: opportunity retrospective study of medical charts in China. BMJ 2010;341:c4779.
23. Wenzel RP, Edmond MB. Preparing for 2009 H1N1 Influenza. N Engl J Med 2009; 361:1991–3.
24. Belshe RB. Implications of the emergence of a novel H1 influenza virus. N Engl J Med 2009;360(25):2667–8.
25. Arguedas A, Soley C, Lindert K. Responses to 2009 H1N1 vaccine in children 3 to 17 years of age. N Engl J Med 2010;362:370–2.
26. Wichmann O, Stöcker P, Poggensee G, et al. Pandemic influenza A(H1N1) 2009 breakthrough infections and estimates of vaccine effectiveness in Germany 2009-2010. Euro Surveill 2010;15(18). Available at: http://www.eurosurveillance.org/ViewArticle.aspx?Articleid=19561. Accessed April 4, 2011. pii: 19561.
27. Fiore AE, Uyeki TM, Broder K, et al. Prevention and control of influenza with vaccines. Recommendation of the Advisory Committee on Immunization Practices (ACIP), 2010. MMWR Recomm Rep 2010;59:61.
28. Centers for Disease Control and Prevention. Safety of influenza A (H1N1) 2009 monovalent vaccines—United States, October 1-November 24, 2009. MMWR Morb Mortal Wkly Rep 2009;58:1351–6.
29. Centers for Disease Control and Prevention. Preliminary results: surveillance for Guillain-Barré syndrome after receipt of influenza A (H1N1) 2009 monovalent vaccine—United States, 2009-2010. MMWR Morb Mortal Wkly Rep 2010;59: 657–61.
30. Chan M. H1N1 in post-pandemic period. World Health Organization Media centre. August 10, 2010. Available at: http://www.who.int/mediacentre/news/statements/2010h1n1_vpc_20100810/en/index.html. Accessed April 14, 11.
31. Centers for Disease Control and Prevention. Final estimates for 2009-2010 seasonal influenza and influenza A (H1N1) 2009 monovalent vaccination coverage—United States, August 2009 through May, 2010. Available at: www.cdc.gov/flu/professionals/vaccination/coverage_910estimates.htm. Accessed March 12, 2011. p. 1–5.
32. Centers for Disease Control and Prevention. Seasonal influenza and 2009 H1N1 influenza vaccination coverage among pregnant women—10 states, 2009-10 influenza season. MMWR Morb Mortal Wkly Rep 2010;59:1541–5.
33. Centers for Disease Control and Prevention. Update: influenza activity—United States, August 30, 2009-March 27, 2010, and composition of the 2010 influenza vaccine. MMWR Morb Mortal Wkly Rep 2010;59:423–30.

Cancer Vaccines

Christopher V. Chambers, MD

KEYWORDS

• Cancer • Vaccine • Prophylactic • Therapeutic

Vaccines have the potential to boost the immune system's ability both to prevent the infections that cause some cancers and to help the immune system identify altered or abnormal cells, including cancer cells, in the treatment of other cancers. Preventive, or prophylactic vaccines, work primarily by stimulating the production of antibodies by B cell lymphocytes. These antibodies bind to the targeted microbes and block their ability to cause infection that can lead to cancer. Prophylactic cancer vaccines, which include those directed at hepatitis B virus (HBV) and human papillomavirus (HPV), also work by boosting cellular immunity. In addition, cytotoxic T cells, or so-called killer T cells, are recruited to help kill already infected cells that have been identified by the immune system as altered, or prompt these cells to self-destruct (a process known as apoptosis). Cancer treatment vaccines, which are also referred to as therapeutic vaccines, work by activating B cells and killer T cells and helping them to recognize and act against cancer cells. In some cases, this involves isolating an antigen from cancer cells taken from the affected patient and creating a vaccine to present the antigen back to the patient, thereby stimulating the immune system to attack the cancer. Helper T cells and dendritic cells help activate killer T cells as part of the cellular immune response. There are many therapeutic cancer vaccines currently being evaluated in clinical trials, most of which are given in combination with other forms of cancer therapy. The first cancer treatment vaccine to be approved by the US Food and Drug Administration (FDA) (in 2010) is indicated for use in some men with metastatic prostate cancer.

CANCER PREVENTION VACCINES

Hepatitis B Vaccine

Liver cancer is the third leading cause of cancer-related deaths in the world and the ninth leading cause of cancer deaths in the United States.[1,2] Nearly 80% of all cases are associated with underlying chronic hepatitis B or hepatitis C infection.[3] In the United States, hepatocellular carcinoma (HCC) occurs predominantly in adults, many of whom acquired hepatitis B or C through intravenous drug use. In other parts of the world, such as southeast Asia, where hepatitis B infection is endemic, HCC occurs in persons of all ages, including children. Although epidemiologic evidence

Department of Family and Community Medicine, Jefferson Medical College, Thomas Jefferson University, 1015 Walnut Street, Suite 401, Philadelphia, PA 19107, USA
E-mail address: Christopher.Chambers@jefferson.edu

Prim Care Clin Office Pract 38 (2011) 703–715
doi:10.1016/j.pop.2011.07.008 **primarycare.theclinics.com**
0095-4543/11/$ – see front matter

has established that chronic HBV infections are associated with the development of HCC, the mechanism of oncogenic transformation remains elusive. Multiple studies have implicated a protein known as the HBV X protein (HBX) as playing an important role.[4,5] HBX regulates several cellular signal transduction pathways including those that modulate cell proliferation. HBX also indirectly or directly affects the levels and activities of several other cell cycle regulatory proteins that, working in combination, can induce normally quiescent cells to replicate. This process may help explain why HCC can develop in patients with apparently inactive infection after many years. Treatments for chronic HBV infection and for HCC have not been successful and efforts have focused instead on prevention.

The original hepatitis B vaccine was approved in 1981, making it the first cancer prevention vaccine to be successfully developed and marketed. In 1984, Taiwan launched the world's first universal HBV vaccination program for infants.[6] The effectiveness of the hepatitis B vaccine in preventing HCC in Taiwan has been dramatic and was measurable in children within 2 decades. With the introduction of the universal vaccination program, all newborn infants were given a series of 3 or 4 doses of recombinant hepatitis B vaccine. In addition, infants of highly infectious (positive to the hepatitis B e antigen [HBeAg]) mothers received hepatitis B immunoglobulin within 24 hours of birth. Nearly all eligible infants were vaccinated as part of the program. The overall immunization rate was reported at 97%. After 20 years, the seroprevalence of the hepatitis B surface antigen (HB_SAg) in children declined from 9.8% (prevaccination period) to 0.6%.[7] This decrease in infection was associated with a significant reduction in childhood HCC (**Table 1**). In a 13 year period (1981–1994), the incidence of HCC in children between 6 and 9 years old declined from 0.52/100,000 for children born between 1974 and 1984 to 0.13/100,000 for those born between 1984 and 1986 ($P<.001$). The HCC cases that were not prevented by the vaccine program were subsequently investigated in an evaluation of the program. In more than 90% of the HCC cases, both the affected child and the mother, were HB_SAg-positive in spite of the universal vaccination program. The vaccine failure has been attributed to poor compliance with the 3-shot series, genetic hyporesponsiveness (to the vaccine), and vaccine escape mutants (viruses with enough antigenic changes to avoid immune recognition).[8]

The hepatitis B vaccine has been clearly shown to be an effective, preventive vaccine against HCC. Consequently, all infants are immunized routinely. The duration of the protective effect in healthy individuals is not known and the need for boosters in the at-risk population has not been defined. Adults at high risk because of possible exposure to blood or because of chronic hepatitis C should also be immunized. Booster vaccinations should be considered in some particularly high-risk groups.

HPV INFECTION

Epidemiology

HPV infections are now recognized as the cause of multiple human cancers, most prominently cervical cancer. Worldwide, cervical cancer is the second most common

Table 1
Effect of universal hepatitis B vaccination of infants in Taiwan (1984)

	% HB_SAg-Positive (All Children)	HCC Incidence per 100,000 (6–9 Years Old)
Before 1984	9.8	0.52
After 1984	0.6	0.13

Data from Ni YH, Chen DS. Hepatitis B vaccination in children: the Taiwan experience. Pathol Biol 2010;4:296.

cause of cancer-related deaths in women in underdeveloped countries. In wealthier nations where women are routinely screened for precancerous cervical changes and then treated as necessary, few women develop invasive cancer and even fewer die from the disease. Nonetheless, in the United States, it is estimated that 12,200 women were newly diagnosed with cervical cancer and that 4210 women died of the disease in 2010.[9] The importance of HPV in this disease cannot be overstated. Persistent infection of the cervix with an oncogenic HPV type is now recognized as a necessary precursor to the development of cervical cancer. Careful analysis of pathologic specimens internationally has detected HPV DNA in 99.7% of cancerous cervical lesions.[10] Approximately 40 HPV types infect the genital skin or mucosa. Of these, 15 are considered oncogenic and therefore labeled as high-risk types. The 2 most common oncogenic HPV types associated with cervical cancer are types 16 and 18.

However, the burden of HPV-related cancers encompasses many other sites, both genital and extragenital (**Table 2**).[11] Among the other genital sites, there are nearly 4000 new cases of vulvar cancer and more than 2000 new cases of vaginal cancer diagnosed in the United States annually, half or more of which are caused by HPV.[9] Penile cancer is uncommon among US men with only 1250 new cases in 2010.[9] However, up to 40% of cancers of the penis have oncogenic HPV DNA detected within them.

Anal cancer affects both men and women, with approximately 60% of cases occurring in women. According to the American Cancer Society, it is estimated that approximately 2000 men and more than 3000 women were diagnosed with anal cancer in 2010.[9] The rates of in situ and invasive anal cancer among women seem to be increasing (**Fig. 1**).[12] The reasons for these changes are not known but may be attributable to changes in sexual practices.

There has been an increase in the incidence of oropharyngeal squamous cell carcinoma (OSCC) in adults without a history of alcohol or cigarette use in the past decade. In 2010, there were an estimated 36,540 new cases of OSCC in the United States, with an expected 7880 deaths attributed to these cancers.[9] A recent analysis of these data showed that, although the incidence of squamous cell carcinomas in many of the oral and pharyngeal sites has remained constant or decreased, there has been an increase in the incidence of cancers of the lingual and palatine tonsils, particularly among younger patients.[13] These cancers of the posterior tongue and the tonsils have been increasingly linked to infection with HPV type 16. Thus, the portion of OSCCs related to HPV infection rather than to cigarette and alcohol use has increased, another change in epidemiology that may be the result of changing sexual behaviors (**Fig. 2**).[13]

Acquisition of HPV

HPV is transmitted through microabrasions in the epithelium that may occur during sexual intercourse or other sexual exposure. Consequently, HPV can infect any skin

Table 2
Beyond cervical cancer: the burden of HPV-related cancers

Cancer Site	% HPV-Related
Vulvar	40–51
Vaginal	40–64
Anal	90–93
Penile	36–40
Oropharyngeal	2–63

Data from Chaturvedi A. Beyond cervical cancer: burden of other HPV- related cancers among men and women. J Adolesc Health 2010;46:20.

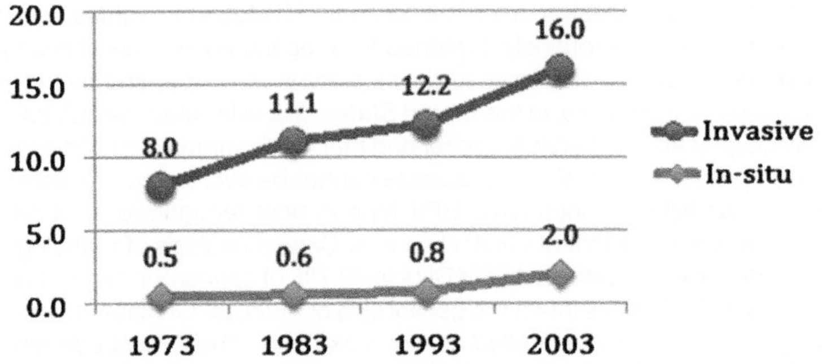

Fig. 1. Age-adjusted incidence rates (per 1,000,000 persons) of in situ and invasive anal cancer among women, 1973 to 2003.

or mucosal surface that it comes in contact with, including the cervical, vaginal, penile, and oropharyngeal epithelium. Of the anatomic locations that can be infected with HPV, 88% of HPV-related cancers worldwide occur in the cervix.[14]

HPV is the most common sexually transmitted infection among adolescents, and approximately 50% of women contract the infection within the first 3 years after onset of sexual activity.[15,16] The peak prevalence of HPV infection is observed in women less than 24 years of age, a finding that may result from an increased susceptibility in the years following sexual debut.[17] There seems to be a smaller secondary minor peak in HPV prevalence in women aged 30 to 39 years.[18] Older women also have a higher risk of persistent infection and disease progression. For this reason, the long-term protection from HPV vaccination is important. The overall prevalence of infection among American girls and women aged 14–59 years is estimated at 26.8% (**Fig. 3**).[17] However, most HPV infections are transient; 70% of infections are cleared naturally by the immune system within 12 months, increasing to approximately 90% at 24 months after infection.[19] However, a small percentage of women develop persistent HPV infections, defined as detection of the same HPV type at least 2 consecutive

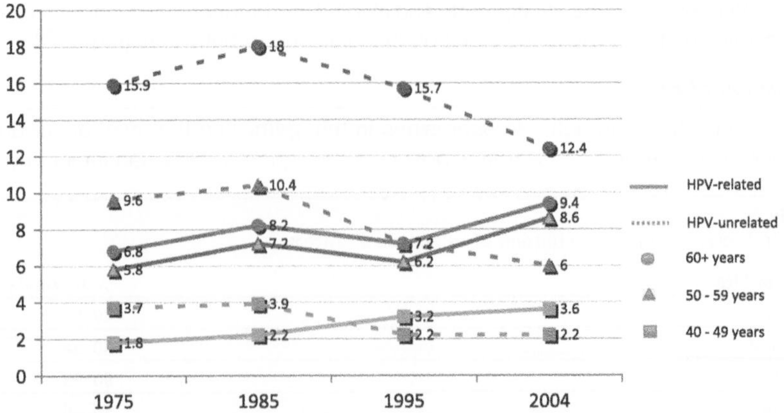

Fig. 2. Incidence of HPV-related and HPV-unrelated OSCCs per 100,000 person years. (*Data from* Chaturverdi A, Engels E, Anderson W, et al. Incidence trends for human papillomavirus-related and-unrelated oral squamous cell carcinomas in the United States. J Clin Oncol 2008;28:612.)

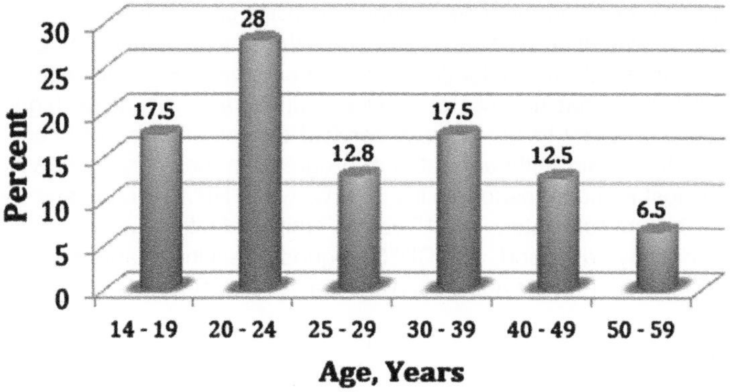

Fig. 3. Point prevalence oncogenic HPV, by age. (*Data from* Dunne EF, Unger ER, Sternberg M, et al. Prevalence of HPV infection among females in the United States. JAMA 2007; 297(8):813–9.)

times in a specified period, typically 6–12 months. At present, there is no method to accurately predict which infections will persist versus those that will eventually resolve spontaneously.

HPV: Pathogenesis and Evasion of the Immune System

HPV infects the basal cells of the cervical transformation zone. The transformation zone is an area of rapid cellular proliferation where columnar epithelium is replaced by squamous epithelium via the process of squamous metaplasia. The increased rate of cellular proliferation during adolescence is believed to contribute to the higher vulnerability to HPV infection in this age group.[20] In the presence of oncogenic HPV infection, squamous metaplasia can develop into precancerous lesions.

The viral life cycle of HPV occurs entirely within the epithelium, mimicking the natural life cycle of a cervical basal cell.[21] This location allows the virus to avoid host immune responses by a variety of methods. First, because HPV infection lacks a systemic viremic phase, an effective immune response to natural infection by HPV must be generated locally at the site of infection. However, the host's antibody response to natural infection is blunted.[22] Second, the infected epithelial cells do not die prematurely, thereby avoiding an inflammatory response. Third, HPV is able to downregulate the expression of proteins involved in the immune response and resistance to infection. Through these strategies, HPV is able to prolong evasion of the host's immune defenses.

As a result, only about 50% of the women who are able to clear HPV infection naturally develop detectable levels of antibodies against HPV.[23] These levels are generally low and may not consistently protect against future reinfection. Naturally induced antibody responses to HPV-16 and HPV-18 are less effective at preventing infection with the same HPV type compared with naive (ie, seronegative) women. In addition, because antibody production is specific to each HPV type, an individual seropositive for one HPV type is susceptible to infections caused by other types.

Progression of Cervical Disease: From Infection to Precancerous Lesions and Cancer

Once an infection is established by an oncogenic HPV type, expression of viral oncogenes allows for the development of precancerous lesions.[24] Histologically, lesions are classified as cervical intraepithelial neoplasia (CIN) grades 1, 2, and 3, reflecting the depth of involvement of dysplastic cells within the cervical epithelium. CIN 1 refers to low-grade lesions indicating infection with a nononcogenic HPV type or an infection with a high-risk type that has not progressed. CIN 2 and 3 indicate higher-grade lesions with a propensity to progress to cervical cancer because of infection from an oncogenic HPV strain. Although rates of progression may vary by HPV type and the individual host immune response, the time between HPV infection and the emergence of CIN 3 is approximately 7 to 15 years.[25] Initial infections usually occur in late adolescence or early adulthood, with CIN 3 diagnosis peaking at approximately 25 to 30 years of age and a median age at cervical cancer diagnosis of 48 years.[26]

HPV VACCINE

Effective cervical cancer prevention programs have been implemented in developed countries with widespread use of the Papanicolaou (Pap) test. The costs associated with screening and treatment of HPV-related diseases are estimated at approximately 6 billion dollars annually in the United States.[27,28] The Pap test detects the development of precancerous cervical lesions and, as such, is a form of secondary prevention of cervical cancer. In contrast, HPV vaccination prevents the initial infection of the most common oncogenic HPV types associated with cervical cancer. Thus, vaccination against oncogenic HPV is considered the primary form of cervical cancer prevention. Current HPV vaccines prevent infection from oncogenic types 16 and 18, which together account for 70% of cervical cancer cases worldwide (**Fig. 4**). One HPV vaccine also provides protection against genital warts caused by nononcogenic HPV types 6 and 11. Vaccination is most effective when administered to women naive to infection with HPV (typically before sexual debut, although sexual activity does not necessarily affirm HPV exposure).

Clinical trials of the HPV vaccines have shown greater than 95% protection against persistent infection (defined as finding the same HPV type in cervicovaginal secretions on 2 successive pelvic examinations by any of the HPV types included in the vaccine for subjects who have received all 3 shots in the series). As mentioned earlier, persistent infection is a necessary step in the development of cervical cancer.[29,30] The true meaningful end point of the vaccine's efficacy is its ability to prevent cervical

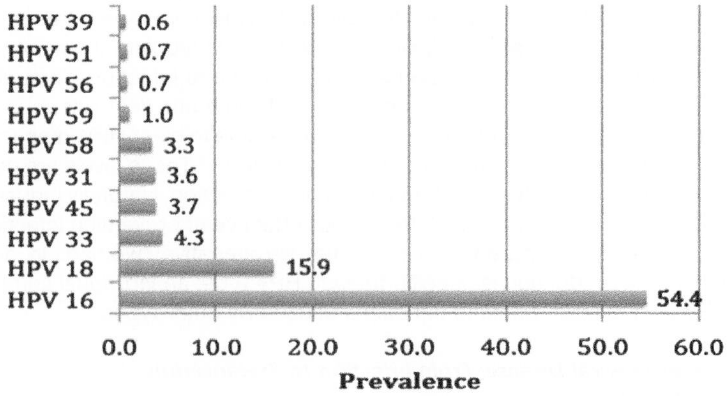

Fig. 4. Oncogenic HPV types and cervical cancer. (*Data from* Smith JS, Lindsay L, Hoots B, et al. Human Papillomavirus type distribution in invasive cervical cancer and high grade cervical lesions: a meta-analysis update. Int J Cancer 2007;121:621–32.)

neoplasia. For ethical reasons, girls and women who develop severe dysplasia in trials receive interventional treatment before they can develop invasive cancer. Therefore, the end points in most trials have been CIN 2 or greater. Although the study populations in the various trials reported for the 2 available vaccines are not exactly comparable, both the bivalent and quadrivalent vaccine have efficacy of greater than 93% against CIN 2 or greater caused by HPV-16 or 18 (**Table 3**).[31,32]

Because as much as 30% of cervical cancer is caused by types other than HPV-16 and HPV-18, it is important to know whether the currently available vaccines protect against neoplasia caused by other HPV types. There is similarity between other HPV types on the phylogenetic tree, so some cross-protection is theoretically possible (**Fig. 5**).[33] Although the numbers are small, both vaccines have shown some cross-protection against oncogenic types other than HPV-16 and HPV-18. The bivalent vaccine, in particular, has shown efficacy against other high-risk types (**Table 4**).[34,35]

Expanded HPV Vaccine Indications

The mucosal epithelium of perianal tissue is histologically analogous to cervical epithelium. It is, therefore, not surprising that most anal cancer is related to infection with the oncogenic HPV types 16 and 18 and that anal warts are caused by infection with HPV types 6 and 11. In late 2010, the quadrivalent HPV vaccine received FDA approval for the prevention of anal cancer caused by HPV types 16 and 18 and for the prevention of anal intraepithelial neoplasia (AIN), including anal warts, caused by HPV types 6, 11, 16, and 18, in people from 9 to 26 years of age. Men who have sex with men (MSMs) may particularly benefit from vaccination. At this time, there are no data regarding the use of the HPV vaccine to prevent oropharyngeal cancers.

Antibody Responses to HPV Vaccination

The mechanism by which HPV vaccines provide protection has not been clearly established. As discussed previously, natural infection with HPV is localized, limited to the basal layer of the epithelium, and never results in a systemic viremia.[21] Consequently, serum levels of neutralizing antibodies after infection are typically low, if detectable, and not a reliable indicator of immunity. This localized infection often

Table 3
Bivalent versus quadrivalent HPV vaccine efficacy against CIN 2+

Vaccine	Vaccine		Placebo		Vaccine Efficacy	
HPV Type	N	Cases	N	Cases	%	Confidence Interval
Bivalent						
HPV-16/18	7344	4	7312	56	93	80, 98
HPV-16		2		46	96	83, 100
HPV-18		2		15	87	40, 99
Quadrivalent						
HPV-16/18	7738	2	7714	100	98	93, 100
HPV-16		2		81	98	91, 100
HPV-18		0		29	100	87, 100

Data from Paavonen J, Naud P, Salmeron J, et al. Efficacy of human papillomavirus (HPV)-16/18 AS04-adjuvanted vaccine against cervical infection and precancer caused by oncogenic HPV types (PATRICIA): final analysis of a double-bind, randomized study in young women. Lancet 2009;374(9686):301–14; and Kjaer S, Sigurdsson K, Iversen O, et al. A pooled analysis of continued prophylactic efficacy of quadrivalent human papillomavirus (Types 6/11/16/18) vaccine against high-grade cervical and external genital lesions. Institute of Cancer Epidemiology; 2009. p. 1–3.

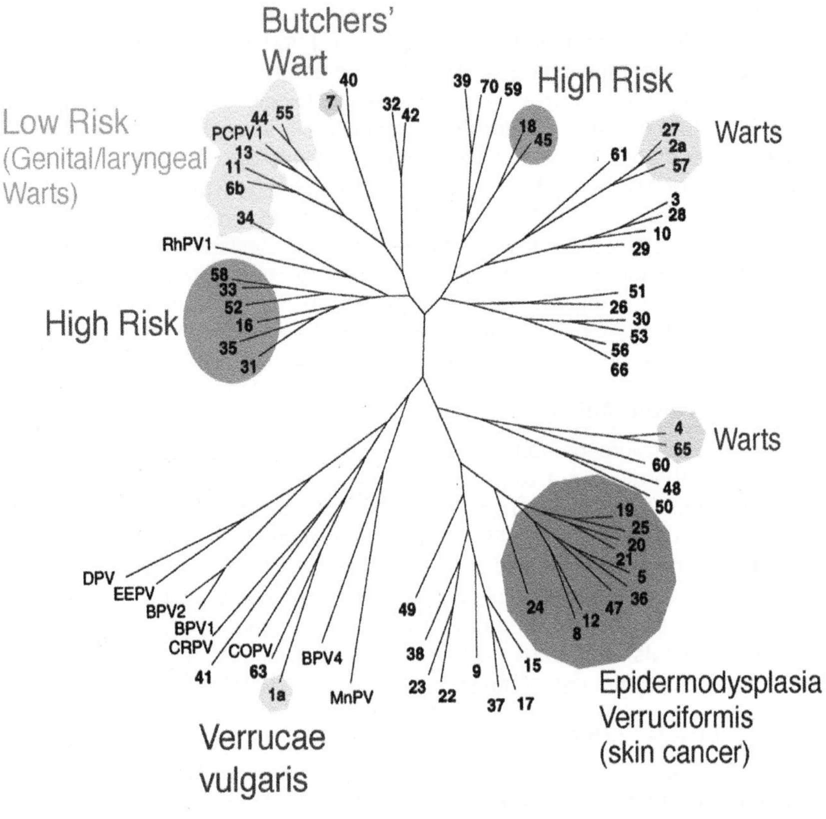

Fig. 5. HPV phylogenetic tree. (*From* Burns J, Maitland N. Human papillomaviruses and cancer. England: Microbiology Today. August 2005. p. 116–20; used with permission from the journal.)

Table 4
Efficacy against CIN2+ caused by nonvaccine oncogenic HPV types

Vaccine			Vaccine Efficacy	
HPV Type	Vaccine Cases	Control Cases	%	Confidence Interval
Bivalent				
31/33/35/52/58	16	47	66	37, 83
31/33/35/39/51/52/56/58/59	20	63	68	46, 82
Quadrivalent				
31/33/35/52/58	44	69	35	4, 57
31/33/35/39/45/51/52/56/58/59	62	93	33	6, 52

Data from Bonanni P, Boccalini S, Bechini A. Progress in the research on HPV vaccination: updates from the 25th International Papillomarvirus Conference in Malmo, Sweden, 2009. J Prev Med Hyg 2009;50:131–4; and Brown D, Kjaer S, Sigurdsson K, et al. The impact of quadrivalent human papillomavirus (HPV; Types 6, 11, 16, and 18) L1 virus-like particle vaccine on infection and disease due to oncogenic nonvaccine HPV types in generally HPV-naïve women aged 16–26 years. J Infect Dis 2008;199(7):926–35.

results in immune tolerance, allowing a low-grade, persistent infection to propagate for years or longer.[22] In contrast, the HPV vaccines elicit high titers of anti-L1 viruslike particle (VLP) (neutralizing) antibodies that far exceed those of natural infection and persist for years.[35] It has been hypothesized that the primary mechanism of protection of HPV vaccines is by producing neutralizing antibodies that prevent entry of the virus into the basal layer of epithelium. Although there have been too few vaccine failures to be able to determine an unequivocal immune correlate of protection,[36] the World Health Organization has stated that the major basis of protection against HPV is primarily meditated through the presence of neutralizing antibodies at the genital mucosa.[37]

Duration of Protection

The minimum anti-HPV titer that confers protective efficacy has not yet been determined. For quadrivalent vaccine, antibody titers have been reported for up to 5 years after vaccination.[29] These data show that more than 99% of women were seropositive for anti–HPV-16 and anti–HPV-18 antibodies at month 7 (ie, 1 month following the third vaccine dose). Geometric mean titers (GMTs) of neutralizing antibodies for vaccine HPV types peaked at month 7, declined through month 24, and stabilized at levels more than the baseline until month 60. For the bivalent vaccine, GMTs for both HPV-16 and HPV-18 peaked at month 7 and subsequently reached a plateau that was sustained for 6.4 years.[38] More than 98% of subjects remained seropositive for both HPV-16 and HPV-18 antibodies throughout this period. The immunoassays used to analyze each vaccine are unique, and therefore results across vaccines cannot be compared.

Long-term efficacy data from phase II studies provide further evidence of the duration of protection following vaccination against HPV. The quadrivalent vaccine has shown 100% efficacy (95% confidence interval [CI]12.3, 100.0) against CIN of any grade, adenocarcinoma in situ (AIS), vulvar or vaginal neoplasia of any severity related to HPV types 16 and 18, and genital warts related to vaccine HPV types 6 and 11 at 5 years among subjects in the per-protocol population (naive to the relevant HPV types at baseline).[29] The bivalent vaccine has shown 100% efficacy (98.67% CI 28.4, 100.0) against CIN 2/3 or AIS associated with HPV-16 or HPV-18 at 6.4 years of follow-up (mean 5.9 years) in subjects naive to current oncogenic HPV infection or prior exposure to HPV-16 and HPV-18 at the time of vaccination. The same cohort also showed 100% efficacy (98.67% CI 74.4, 100) against 12-month persistent infection with HPV-16 or HPV-18.[38]

Based on the available efficacy and immunogenicity data (with up to 6.4 years of follow-up), mathematical models have been used to estimate the duration of protection following vaccination with the bivalent vaccine in girls and women aged 15 to 25 years. These models showed that vaccine-induced levels of antibodies against HPV-16 and HPV-18 may remain significantly higher than those produced in response to natural infection for 20 years (see **Fig. 2**).

For both vaccines, the magnitude of the immune response seems to be related to the age of the recipient. In immunobridging studies conducted in younger girls, those administered the quadrivalent vaccine (aged 9–15 years) or the bivalent vaccine (aged 10–14 years) showed seroconversion rates against HPV-16 and HPV-18 greater than 99%.[29,38] In studies for the respective HPV vaccines, the GMTs of these younger girls were roughly twofold higher compared with those immunized at 15 years of age or older. In theory, the higher titers observed in younger girls may result in longer persistence of neutralizing antibodies, and therefore a longer duration of protection against HPV disease.

The Clinical Importance of Duration of Protection

According to current recommendations, the HPV vaccine should be administered to all girls and women between the ages of 9 and 26 years. The emphasis on vaccination of girls between 11 and 12 years old is because the highest vaccine efficacy has been observed in HPV-naive women, and that HPV is often first acquired in younger girls. Among those previously exposed to HPV, immunity following natural infection is unreliable, and the risk of reinfection remains.[23] Although neither HPV vaccine is therapeutic for those currently infected, the vaccines may be able to prevent reinfection in women previously infected with one of the HPV types included in the vaccine but who are currently clear of the infection.[39]

Although the peak of prevalence of HPV infection occurs in women in their early 20s, the peak prevalence of CIN 2 and CIN 3 occurs between the ages of 25 and 29 years. Cervical cancer does not typically occur until women are in their early 40s. Taken together with evidence that HPV infection later in life is associated with higher rates of persistence and progression, these findings underscore the need for effective vaccines that provide long-term protection against the disease. Ideally, prophylactic HPV vaccines should confer protection against HPV throughout a woman's lifetime. Therefore, it is important for HPV vaccines to deliver long-term protection following vaccine administration. It is not yet known whether the currently recommended vaccines will provide protection throughout a woman's reproductive life or whether boosters will be needed. Studies are ongoing to address this question.

CANCER TREATMENT VACCINES

Theory

Cancer vaccines have been studied as potential treatment of different types of cancer for more than 2 decades. Cancer vaccines have been developed using whole cancer cells, parts of cells, and purified cancer antigen. Although there are many different formulations for these vaccines, the desired outcome underlying their use is the same, namely to stimulate the patient's immune system to identify and kill tumor cells.

Tumor cell vaccines are made from cancer cells that are inactivated and then infused back into the patient. Tumor cell vaccines can be autologous (ie, made from cells from the cancer of the patient into whom they will later be injected) or allogeneic (made from cancer cells from someone other than the patient who is being treated). Autologous cancer vaccines are more specific to the individual but more expensive to prepare. Tumor cell vaccines have been developed for use in more than 10 cancers including breast, prostate, melanoma, and lung cancer.

Cancer Vaccine Efficacy

In clinical trials, cancer vaccines have typically been given along with chemotherapy and other treatments. However, it has been difficult to show any measurable benefit from the addition of immunotherapy in most trials. The reasons for this are probably complex. Chemotherapeutic agents are cytotoxic and effective treatment can result in clinical regression within a matter of weeks. However, cancer vaccines rely on stimulating humoral and cellular immunity, a process that may require months before becoming fully activated. Therefore, it is possible that the cancer being treated could continue to progress for a significant period of time following the initiation of immunotherapy before stabilizing and then regressing. Second, chemotherapy often weakens the immune system and, in particular, the cellular response that is required for cancer vaccines to be effective.[40]

Another possible explanation for the ineffectiveness of cancer vaccines to date is that factors within the local tumor environment may inhibit the immune system. Recent evidence suggests that stromal cells within certain tumors may produce a protein that suppresses the immune response and limits the potential of cancer vaccine or other forms of immunotherapy.[40] This protein, fibroblast activation protein α (FAP), seems to play a major role in allowing the tumor to grow. To determine whether FAP-expressing stromal cells were contributing to a tumor's resistance to vaccination, a group of researchers used a transgenic mouse model that allowed them to destroy FAP-expressing cells. When these cells were destroyed in tumors of mice with lung cancers (<2% of the tumor cells express FAP), the tumors began to rapidly regress. If similar immune suppressive factors are found in humans, cancer vaccines may become a more important part of cancer treatment in the future.

An FDA-approved Cancer Vaccine

In 2010, the FDA approved the first therapeutic cancer vaccine for use in some men with metastatic prostate cancer.[41] This vaccine, which is called sipuleucel-T, is indicated for men with advanced prostate cancer that is no longer responding to hormonal therapy, or so-called hormone-resistant or castration-resistant cancer. In trials, sipuleucel-T improved 3-year survival by approximately 40% compared with placebo (32.1% vs 23%) with a median improvement in overall survival of 4.1 months (25.8 months vs 21.7 months).

Sipuleucel-T is an autologous vaccine, customized for each individual patient. Before treatment, prospective patients undergo leukapheresis to isolate antigen-presenting cells (APCs) from their blood. The APCs include dendritic cells and macrophages that present antigens to the patient's immune system to elicit an augmented immune reaction. The APCs are cultured with an antigen (prostate acid phosphatase) in a laboratory and then returned to the patients' treating physician. During a period of 4 to 6 weeks, hundreds of millions of APCs are infused during 3 treatments. Subsequent rounds require the same manufacturing process.

REFERENCES

1. Parkin DM, Bray F, Ferlay J, et al. Global cancer statistics, 2002. CA Cancer J Clin 2005;55:74.
2. Alterkruse SF, McGlynn KA, Reichman ME. Hepatocellular carcinoma incidence, mortality, and survival trends in the United States from 1975 to 2005. J Clin Oncol 2009;27:1485.
3. Perz JF, Armstrong GL, Farrington LA. The contributions of hepatitis B virus and hepatitis C virus infections to cirrhosis and primary liver cancer worldwide. J Hepatol 2006;45:529.
4. Hong T, Naoki O, Shuichi K. Molecular functions and biological roles of hepatitis B virus X protein. Cancer Sci 2006;97:977.
5. Gearhart T, Bouchard M. The hepatitis B virus X protein modulates hepatocyte proliferation pathways to stimulate viral replication. J Virol 2010;6:2675.
6. Chang MH, Chen CJ, Lai MS. Universal hepatitis B vaccination in Taiwan and the incidence of hepatocellular carcinoma in children. N Engl J Med 1997;26:1855.
7. Ni YH, Chen DS. Hepatitis B vaccination in children: the Taiwan experience. Pathol Biol 2010;4:296.
8. Chang MH, You SL, Chen CJ. Decreased incidence of hepatocellular carcinoma in hepatitis B vaccines: a 20-year follow-up study. J Natl Cancer Inst 2009;19:1348.
9. Estimated new cancer cases and deaths by sex for all sites. Available at: www.cancer.org/acs/groups/content/@40epidemiologysurveillance. Accessed February 20, 2011.

10. Walboomers JM, Jacobs MV, Manos MM, et al. Human papillomavirus is a necessary cause of invasive cervical cancer worldwide. J Pathol 1999;189:12.
11. Chaturvedi A. Beyond cervical cancer: burden of other HPV-related cancers among men and women. J Adolesc Health 2010;46:20.
12. Yurri B, Shvetsov B, Hernandez K, et al. Duration and clearance of anal human papillomavirus (HPV) infection among women: the Hawaii HPV cohort study. Clin Infect Dis 2009;48:536–46.
13. Chaturverdi A, Engels E, Anderson W, et al. Incidence trends for human papillomavirus-related and -unrelated oral squamous cell carcinomas in the United States. J Clin Oncol 2008;28:612.
14. Parkin D. The global health burden of infection-associated cancers in the year 2002. Int J Cancer 2006;118(12):3030–44.
15. Collins SI, Mazloomzadeh S, Winter H, et al. Proximity of first intercourse to menarche and the risk of human papillomavirus infection: a longitudinal study. Int J Cancer 2005;1143(3):498–500.
16. Winer RL, Lee SK, Hughes JP, et al. Genital human papillomavirus infection: incidence and risk factors in a cohort of female university students. Am J Epidemiol 2003;157(3):218–26.
17. Dunne EF, Unger ER, Sternberg M, et al. Prevalence of HPV infection among females in the United States. JAMA 2007;297(8):813–9.
18. Castle PE, Schiffman M, Herrero R, et al. A prospective study of age trends in cervical human papillomavirus acquisition and persistence in Guanacaste, Costa Rica. J Infect Dis 2005;191(11):1808–16.
19. Ho GY, Bierman R, Beardsley L, et al. Natural history of cervicovaginal papillomavirus infection in young women. N Engl J Med 1998;338(7):423–8.
20. Moscicki AB, Schiffman M, Kjaer S, et al. Chapter 5: updating the natural history of HPV and anogenital cancer. Vaccine 2006;24(Suppl 3):S42–51.
21. Stanley M. Immune responses to human papillomavirus. Vaccine 2006;24(Suppl 1): S16–22.
22. Tindle RW. Immune evasion in human papillomavirus-associated cervical cancer. Nat Rev Cancer 2002;2(1):59–65.
23. Viscidi RP, Schiffman M, Hildesheim A, et al. Seroreactivity to human papillomavirus (HPV) types 16, 18, or 31 and risk of subsequent HPV infection: results from a population-based study in Costa Rica. Cancer Epidemiol Biomarkers Prev 2004;13(2):324–7.
24. Einstein MH, Schiller JT, Viscidi RP, et al. Clinician's guide to human papillomavirus immunology: knowns and unknowns. Lancet Infect Dis 2009;9(6):347–56.
25. Bosch FX, de Sanjose S. Chapter 1: Human papillomavirus and cervical cancer—burden and assessment of causality. J Natl Cancer Inst Monogr 2003;(31):3–13.
26. National Cancer Institute. SEER Stat Fact Sheets: Cancer of the cervix uteri. Available at: http://seer.cancer.gov/statfacts/html/cervix.html. Accessed October 2, 2008.
27. Insinga RP, Dasbach EJ, Elbasha EH. Assessing the annual economic burden of preventing and treating anogenital human papillomavirus-related disease in the U.S.: analytic framework and review of the literature. Pharmacoeconomics 2005; 23(11):1107–22.
28. Chesson HW, Ekwueme DU, Saraiya M, et al. Cost effectiveness of human papillomavirus vaccination in the United States. Emerg Infect Dis 2008;14(2):244–51.
29. Smith JS, Lindsay L, Hoots B, et al. Human papillomavirus type distribution in invasive cervical cancer and high grade cervical lesions: a meta-analysis update. Int J Cancer 2007;121:621–32.
30. CERVARIX prescribing information. Rixensart (Belgium): GlaxoSmithKline; 2009.

31. Paavonen J, Naud P, Salmeron J, et al. Efficacy of human papillomavirus (HPV)-16/18 AS04-adjuvanted vaccine against cervical infection and precancer caused by oncogenic HPV types (PATRICIA): final analysis of a double-bind, randomized study in young women. Lancet 2009;374(9686):301–14.
32. Kjaer S, Sigurdsson K, Iversen O, et al. A pooled analysis of continued prophylactic efficacy of quadrivalent human papillomavirus (Types 6/11/16/18) vaccine against high-grade cervical and external genital lesions. Denmark: Institute of Cancer Epidemiology; 2009. p. 1–3.
33. Burns J, Maitland N. Human papillomaviruses and cancer. Microbiology Today. August 2005. p. 116–20.
34. Bonanni P, Boccalini S, Bechini A. Progress in the research on HPV vaccination: updates from the 25th International Papillomavirus Conference in Malmo, Sweden, 2009. J Prev Med Hyg 2009;50:131–4.
35. Brown D, Kjaer S, Sigurdsson K, et al. The impact of quadrivalent human papillomavirus (HPV; types 6, 11, 16, and 18) L1 virus-like particle vaccine on infection and disease due to oncogenic nonvaccine HPV types in generally HPV-naïve women aged 16-26 years. J Infect Dis 2008;199(7):926–35.
36. Koutsky LA, Harper DM. Chapter 13: Current findings from prophylactic HPV vaccine trials. Vaccine 2006;24(Suppl 3):S3/114–21.
37. Human papillomavirus (HPV) vaccine background paper. Canberra: WHO; 2008. Available at: http://www.google.com/webhp?sourceid=toolbar-instant&hl=en&ion=1&qscrl=1&nord=1&rlz=1T4ADRA_enUS432US434#sclient=psy&hl=en&qscrl=1&nord=1&rlz=1T4ADRA_enUS432US434&site=webhp&source=hp&q=human%20papillomavirus%20vaccine%20background%20paper%20WHO&aq=0n&aqi=q-n1&aql=&oq=&pbx=1&fp=68b3f9ae28a95316&ion=1&ion=1&bav=on.2,or.r_gc.r_pw.&fp=68b3f9ae28a95316&ion=1&biw=793&bih=560. Accessed July 20, 2011.
38. GARDASIL prescribing information. Whitehouse Station (NJ): Merck; 2009.
39. Fraser C, Tomassini JE, Xi L, et al. Modeling the long-term antibody response of a human papillomavirus (HPV) virus-like particle (VLP) type 16 prophylactic vaccine. Vaccine 2007;25(21):4324–33.
40. Kraman M, Bambrough P, Arnold J, et al. Suppression of antitumor immunity by fibroblast activation protein: expressing stromal cells. Science 2010;330:827–30.
41. FDA approves first therapeutic cancer vaccine. Available at: www.cancer.gov/ncicacerbulletin/050410/page2. Accessed April 10, 2011.

Vaccination Refusal: Ethics, Individual Rights, and the Common Good

Jason L. Schwartz, MBE, AM[a,*], Arthur L. Caplan, PhD[b]

KEYWORDS

• Vaccination • Ethics • Risk • Decision making • Public health

Primary care physicians and other health care providers encounter many challenges related to the administration of vaccines in their practices. Despite the remarkable achievements of vaccination programs in eliminating many vaccine-preventable diseases in the United States and reducing the incidence of others, the continued success of vaccination is threatened by a spectrum of interconnected social and political concerns. Chief among these obstacles is the apparent recent increase in hesitancy and outright resistance to the recommended vaccination schedule by some parents and patients. These attitudes present challenges that are likely to be experienced increasingly by primary care physicians as more vaccines are recommended for adolescents and adults.

In this article, the authors review the spectrum of patient or parental attitudes that may be described as types of vaccine refusal, explore related ethical considerations in the context of the doctor-patient relationship and public health, and evaluate the possible responses of physicians when encountering resistance to vaccination recommendations. The related topic of reluctance by health care workers to receive vaccines personally, particularly annual influenza vaccination, is also examined.

POTENTIAL CAUSES OF VACCINE HESITANCY

Recent controversies regarding vaccine safety have contributed to a surge in information available to parents and providers about vaccines and vaccine-preventable

This work was supported by a grant from The Greenwall Foundation.
The authors have nothing to disclose.
[a] Department of History and Sociology of Science, Center for Bioethics, University of Pennsylvania, 3401 Market Street, Suite 320, Philadelphia, PA 19104, USA
[b] Department of Medical Ethics, Center for Bioethics, University of Pennsylvania, 3401 Market Street, Suite 320, Philadelphia, PA 19104, USA
* Corresponding author.
E-mail address: jlschwa2@mail.med.upenn.edu

Prim Care Clin Office Pract 38 (2011) 717–728
doi:10.1016/j.pop.2011.07.009 primarycare.theclinics.com
0095-4543/11/$ – see front matter

diseases. The quality and accuracy of this information varies widely, particularly on the Internet. Distinguishing reputable resources among these materials can be challenging for members of the public.[1] Of particular concern are allegations linking routinely administered vaccines to a variety of chronic and acute medical conditions.

The most widely publicized vaccine safety controversy is the now-discredited association between vaccines and rising autism rates, a theory popularized by British physician Dr Andrew Wakefield in 1998.[2] Despite a large and growing body of scientific evidence rejecting the link between vaccines and autism, the debate persists, in part due to a vocal cohort of activists led by celebrities and a small number of health care providers who reject the consensus of the global medical and scientific communities.

The alleged link between vaccines and autism is the most prominent example of the spectrum of theories in which vaccine components, specific vaccines, the timing of their administration, or interactions between them are alleged to cause adverse events beyond the limited vaccine-associated risks known to exist. As evidence mounts rejecting the vaccine-autism hypothesis, critics of vaccine safety have directed increasing attention to the total numbers of vaccines and vaccine doses recommended by the Centers for Disease Control and Prevention (CDC), American Academy of Pediatrics (AAP), and American Academy of Family Physicians (AAFP).[3] Some critics of contemporary vaccine policy allege that the various vaccine antigens—particularly those administered simultaneously—interact in harmful ways not recognized by the mainstream medical community.[4]

Theories about vaccine safety deficiencies circulate widely on the Internet, where networks of parents share resources, theories, and reports that appear to validate their concerns. Passionate and articulate representatives of this community regularly appear in popular media coverage of vaccine safety. These factors contribute to the current atmosphere of doubt and anxiety regarding the value of vaccines, including among the large percentage of the public not actively engaged in these debates.

The unambiguous rulings of the Omnibus Autism Proceeding (OAP) rejecting several theories linking vaccines to autism, as well as the disciplinary action taken against Andrew Wakefield in the United Kingdom, may help to explain an apparent shift in media coverage of vaccine safety debates within the past few years.[5] To the dismay of the public health community, media coverage had previously given comparable attention to both proponents and critics of vaccine policy, despite the clear differences in the composition and perceived credibility of each group. Coverage since the OAP decisions has taken a noticeably more skeptical view of vaccine safety critics. A primary theme of this coverage has been examining why debates have persisted despite overwhelming evidence in favor of the safety of vaccines and a clear consensus among public health, medical, and scientific organizations.[6]

Whereas the risks of vaccines—both real and alleged—are readily visible through those individuals who believe vaccines are the cause of their or their child's medical conditions, the benefits of vaccines for individuals and communities are far more difficult to observe. It is often stated that vaccines are "victims of their own success," meaning that the diseases that vaccines prevent have become exceedingly rare in the United States as a result of successful vaccination programs. Many parents and younger physicians have no first-hand awareness of the perils of vaccine-preventable diseases that only a generation ago caused vast suffering and death. Public health officials stress that continued high vaccination rates are critical to ongoing prevention of these diseases, but recognizing the direct and indirect benefits of vaccination may be difficult for parents and providers alike. Recent outbreaks of pertussis and other diseases among unvaccinated populations may unfortunately be making the ongoing risks of vaccine-preventable diseases more visible.[7]

While the recent apparent shift in media attention regarding vaccination may in time alter overall public perceptions of the risks and benefits of vaccines, primary care physicians and other health care providers are currently likely to encounter at least 3 distinct types of patients or parents with reservations regarding vaccines. These groups are:

1. Individuals who have no specific objections to vaccines but are concerned because of the emotional, fervent rhetoric that they have encountered in the media and elsewhere
2. Individuals concerned about specific vaccines or the recommended vaccination schedule who prefer a modified approach to vaccination
3. Individuals with objections to all vaccines without exception, including those with religious or "philosophical" reasons for this position.

Each of these groups presents unique challenges for primary care physicians and raises important ethical considerations deserving of attention.

INDIVIDUAL DECISION MAKING AND PUBLIC HEALTH

Patients and parents bring a broad range of perspectives and attitudes regarding vaccines to their health care providers. Simple classifications such as "pro-vaccine" and "anti-vaccine" fail to appreciate the spectrum of opinions that exist about vaccination and the distinct responses required from physicians. Vaccine hesitancy is distinct from vaccine refusal, and care should be taken in all cases to understand the scope of any concerns, their source, and the responses that are warranted.

While vocal critics of United States vaccination policy appear prominently in popular coverage of vaccine safety controversies, data from the CDC National Immunization Survey indicate that vaccination rates for nearly all vaccines are very high.[8] Despite more than a decade of sustained attention to the alleged risks of vaccination, an overwhelming majority of the American public still believes in the importance of vaccines. However, recent trends reveal challenges to this foundation of support, as rates of nonmedical exemptions to state vaccination requirements are increasing nationwide and are particularly concerning in select communities.[9] Surveys of parental attitudes show a significant amount of uncertainty regarding the risks of vaccination, suggesting that years of allegations regarding vaccine-associated risks have led to doubts among some Americans.

Individual decision making regarding vaccination is particularly complex ethically, because it combines the ethics of medical care as part of the doctor-patient relationship with the ethics of public health. Unlike virtually all other medical interventions administered by health care providers, the decision to receive a vaccine has consequences not only for the individual patient but for others in the community. When vaccination rates in a community are high, all members receive additional protection against vaccine-preventable disease by means of "herd immunity." Herd immunity is particularly valuable because no vaccine is 100% effective, and some individuals are too young to receive vaccines or cannot do so because of medical contraindications. The vaccination rate necessary to produce herd immunity varies among diseases, but generally ranges from 85% to 90%. Nationwide vaccination rates for most established vaccines are at or above this level, but some communities now fall short, placing all citizens in these areas—both vaccinated and unvaccinated—at increased risk of disease.[10]

The community-wide benefits of vaccination are important to public health considerations of vaccination programs, but the administration of vaccines nearly always occurs in the context of a doctor-patient relationship. Vaccination is only one component of long-standing care relationships that address a variety of preventive and therapeutic needs. The success of this relationship depends on mutual trust, shared respect, full disclosure of information, and open communication between physicians and their patients.

ADDRESSING CONFUSION AND UNCERTAINTY

Of the 3 types of vaccine-hesitant individuals, the most numerous are those historically supportive of vaccination but with questions about specific vaccines or theories that have been discussed in the media or among friends and family. These kinds of inquiries may create challenges for providers, but they also provide an opportunity to educate and build trust. Earning and preserving this trust will serve both the physician and patient well throughout the duration of the doctor-patient relationship.

Responding to patient or parental inquiries about scientific or safety-related topics in vaccination presents two distinct types of challenges for physicians. The first is the difficulty of remaining up to date on the latest information about vaccine safety and vaccination in general. Public interest in vaccines in recent years means that information about vaccine research or claims of adverse events are disseminated very quickly to the public. Moreover, much of the most controversial claims regarding the risks and benefits of vaccines have not been subject to peer review, or they appear outside of the information sources typically relied on by physicians to stay informed.

Providers should strive to be familiar with the best available information regarding vaccine safety and related topics as well as those theories and allegations receiving significant attention among the public. Familiarity with this information will best equip the physician to answer questions, clarify concerns, and allay uncertainty regarding the risks and benefits of vaccines.

Remaining fully conversant in both the latest verified information regarding vaccines as well as unconfirmed allegations about them is a challenge even for vaccine specialists. For primary care physicians expected to remain up to date on a staggering variety of topics in prevention, diagnosis, and treatment, the challenge of fluency in vaccine-related topics could seem overwhelming. Recognizing the need for accessible materials that synthesize for physicians key information on vaccines, several public and nonprofit institutions produce regularly updated resources highlighting developments in vaccine science and clinical practice.[11,12]

In addition to knowledge deficits that can impede doctor-patient communication regarding vaccination, several practical and logistical considerations may present further challenges. Vaccination has become routine in the United States, in large part because of its long history of success. As a result, the informed consent process for vaccination may often consist of little more than a few brief questions and answers, and the distribution of government-produced Vaccine Information Statements required by federal law.[13] If a more extensive discussion about the relative risks and benefits of vaccines is sought by a patient or his or her parent, scheduling pressures common to primary care physicians and other health care providers may limit the time available for a thoughtful, respectful dialog. Some physician billing programs only compensate for the actual administration of vaccines, presenting a further disincentive for discussion. None of these reasons, however, are adequate justifications for the omission of fully informed consent prior to vaccination. In addition to reflecting a long-standing ethical imperative, physician recommendations have been shown to be highly influential in patient attitudes about vaccines.[14]

ALTERNATIVE VACCINATION SCHEDULES

Whereas some parents or patients are primarily looking for reassurance that their support for vaccines is justified, a second group has explored issues related to vaccine safety and believes that action is warranted. A particular challenge is those patients who prefer a customized approach to the recommended vaccination schedule.[15]

Vaccination schedules like those proposed by "Dr Bob" Sears in his widely read book are described as "compromises," prioritizing vaccines deemed more important while spacing out the full vaccination schedule over a longer period of time than recommended by the CDC, AAP, and AAFP. The intent of spreading out the vaccination schedule is to reduce the number of vaccine doses administered at any one visit, theoretically reducing both the risk of harmful interactions between simultaneously administered vaccines and the burden on the patient's immune system. These theoretical concerns have been extensively studied, and there is no evidence that the timing and spacing of the current recommended vaccination schedule present risks for healthy patients.[16]

The risks of delaying vaccines, however, are far more clearly understood. These risks include the increased likelihood that a multidose vaccination series will not be completed, as a result of the additional office visits required by alternative schedules, and the longer period of time that children lack full protection.[17] Patients who voluntarily delay vaccination also increase the risk of vaccine-preventable diseases in their communities, particularly among those too young or otherwise unable to receive recommended vaccines. In the pediatric population, this is a particular concern for infants and young children attending day-care facilities.

A parent who wishes to deviate from the recommended vaccination schedule presents an opportunity for the physician to understand the specific concerns motivating this preference. Like all policies regarding vaccines, the timing of the recommended schedule reflects a careful assessment of risks and benefits by leaders in public health, pediatrics, and infectious disease. Physicians should help parents compare the known risks that result from delaying vaccination with the hypothesized, unconfirmed risks an alternative schedule aims to mitigate. Physicians might also discuss with parents the many challenges that the immune system of a child faces every day from foods, the environment, and other "natural" sources. With a more complete understanding of the reasons behind the recommended vaccination schedule, the science supporting those recommendations, and the risks that result from additional time with incomplete protection, the preferences of some parents may change.

Requests for alternative vaccination schedules allow physicians to discuss two related and misleading views of contemporary vaccination policy in the United States. The first is that some of the diseases prevented by routinely recommended vaccines protect against trivial maladies incapable of causing serious disease. Varicella is among the diseases mistakenly characterized in this way. Parents who discount varicella vaccination based on recollections of the once-common childhood experience of chickenpox are likely unaware of the significant varicella-related mortality prior to the introduction of the vaccine in the 1990s.[18]

A second common misconception among some parents preferring alternative schedules is that the current recommendations reflect a "one size fits all" approach to vaccination.[19] While the CDC vaccination schedule provides a framework for the timely administration of all recommended vaccines in healthy individuals, supplementary guidance from CDC and medical societies outlines many groups of individuals for whom alternative approaches are warranted. These groups include those with autoimmune diseases, transplant recipients, and pregnant women, among others. The evidence-based schedule endorsed by CDC and other groups provides more guidance for patients with special health conditions than the most popular alternative schedules.

Despite attempts by physicians to understand parents' preference for alternative vaccination schedules and to clarify the risks and benefits of each approach, not every parent's concerns will be resolved. A continued desire for an alternative vaccination schedule against the recommendation of a physician could be viewed as a type of vaccine refusal. In these cases, the physician or other health care provider should ensure that the individual declining on-time administration of vaccines understands the additional risks associated with that decision. The risks to both the patient and the community should be clearly conveyed, and the potential for conflicts with state school and day-care vaccination requirements should be discussed. Signed declination forms, though not required from parents, are increasingly recommended by medical organizations to convey the gravity of the decision to delay vaccination.[20]

Regardless of the specific mechanisms used, the primary responsibility of the physician is to make clear that the decision to delay or defer completion of the recommended vaccination schedule is not the prudent, risk-free compromise suggested by some. Instead, these actions increase the risk of morbidity and mortality for the patient, their peers, and others in their community.

REFUSING RECOMMENDED VACCINES

Parents preferring a nontraditional approach to routine vaccination present difficulties for health care providers, but the unique risks raised by alternative schedules are generally limited to the additional time needed to complete all recommended vaccinations. However, 85% of pediatricians in one survey reported encountering at least one family in their practices that refused vaccines entirely.[21] Those wanting to decline one or more vaccines present far more significant ethical, clinical, and public health challenges. The number of parents nationwide refusing vaccines remains small in absolute terms, but an upward trend is reflected in recent increases in nonmedical exemptions from state school vaccination requirements.[9]

A parental preference to decline recommended vaccines places strains on the doctor-patient relationship, particularly for physicians committed to vaccination as an essential means of disease prevention. For this reason, networks of parents critical of contemporary vaccine policy circulate lists of physicians comfortable with delaying or declining vaccines. These individuals are rather euphemistically described as "vaccine-friendly" physicians.[22]

A patient or parent wishing not to receive vaccines presents the same opportunities for education that occur when alternative schedules are desired. These discussions should be part of a concerted effort to understand the precise reasons why vaccines are being refused. When inaccurate or imprecise information about vaccine safety, effectiveness, or necessity is the primary cause, an informed physician can provide needed and valuable clarifications.

In other cases, concerns about cost may adversely affect one's willingness to receive vaccines. Parents or patients may be unaware of the federal and state programs available to subsidize vaccine costs for uninsured or underinsured children, including the Vaccines for Children program and state programs supported by Section 317 grants.[23] These programs significantly reduce financial obstacles to childhood vaccination in the United States. There are no comparable public-sector vaccine purchase programs for adult vaccination, but several vaccine manufacturers have established patient assistance programs designed to reduce the cost of vaccines for uninsured or underinsured individuals.[24,25]

A third potential source of resistance to vaccines is the temporary pain or discomfort associated with vaccination, particularly for infants and children receiving vaccines by injection. Some parents may be unsettled seeing their child in apparent distress, even if only momentarily. The physician can remind parents that any short-term discomfort related to vaccine administration is clearly outweighed by the long-term protection vaccination provides against illness and possible death. Recommendations from CDC include a range of measures that may help alleviate discomfort, such as distraction, cooling of the injection site, and topical analgesia.[26]

In addition to identifying the precise reasons for vaccine refusal, physicians should consider who is expressing this preference. For children and adolescents without the legal authority to provide consent for medical care, that responsibility generally falls to parents or guardians. Providers, however, are expected to give increasing attention to the preferences and perspectives of children as they mature into adolescence and young adulthood. This ethical concept of assent complements the legal concept of consent.[27] For older children and adolescents, age groups in which vaccination against human papillomavirus (HPV), meningococcus, and influenza are among those recommended, conflicts between the preferences of parents and patients are possible.

Particularly for HPV vaccination, attention has been directed in the medical literature to waiving parental consent requirements, similar to laws in most states permitting minors to provide consent directly for medical care related to sexually transmitted infections and pregnancy.[28] No states have implemented unique consent requirements for HPV or other vaccines to date, but these complexities highlight the need for physicians to view older children and adolescents as developing, active partners in their own health and medical care.

Potential conflicts between parents and children regarding willingness to be vaccinated provide yet another opportunity for the physician to communicate information about the vital role of vaccines in preventive health and the evidence supporting their safety. This dialog and trust is essential to an effective doctor-patient relationship, most especially for adolescents approaching the age when primary legal and personal responsibility for medical treatment and prevention decisions will transition to them alone.

PHYSICIAN RESPONSES TO VACCINE REFUSAL

Similar to patients seeking alternative vaccination schedules, physician communication with parents or patients refusing vaccines may reveal a fundamental difference of opinion unable to be resolved satisfactorily. For minors, legal interventions that provide necessary medical care against parental wishes have not been used for vaccination, nor are they ethically justified in the absence of an outbreak or similar public health emergency. Although the individual and community benefits of vaccination are clear, there is a legal right in the United States to refuse vaccination. Relying on adversarial measures like the courts to promote vaccination in normal circumstances would establish an unfortunate and ultimately harmful atmosphere for the continued public support of vaccination programs.

Physicians are therefore left with two principal alternatives: either to document refusal and continue the doctor-patient relationship or to discharge the patient and direct them to seek care elsewhere. Documenting refusal ensures that the patient or their parent clearly understands the seriousness of that decision. As with alternative schedules, medical organizations provide sample documents that clearly explain the significant, potentially fatal consequences that may result from vaccine refusal.[20]

Physicians should also advise those opting against vaccination of the additional consequences related to state vaccination requirements. Unvaccinated individuals must obtain either a religious exemption (available in all states except for West Virginia and Mississippi) or a personal-belief exemption (also known as a philosophical exemption, available in 21 states) to attend school or day-care facilities.[9] Individuals with exemptions can be excluded from these facilities during outbreaks.

Some physicians believe that continuing care when vaccination is refused may be interpreted as implicitly condoning poor choices. A growing number of physicians endorse ending the doctor-patient relationship as the appropriate response for these patients. In one survey, 39% of pediatricians said they would dismiss a family refusing all vaccinations, and 28% would dismiss a family that refused select vaccines.[21] Dismissing these patients is thought to reflect the gravity of the decision to refuse vaccination. It also has the practical benefit of reducing the number of unvaccinated children in doctors' offices, settings harboring a concentration of patients with increased susceptibility to infection.[29]

The prospect of terminating care for patients who refuse vaccines is part of a larger legal and ethical discourse on the duty to treat and patient abandonment. In general, a physician is legally and ethically obliged to continue to provide care to a patient with whom a relationship has been established unless "that relationship is terminated by the mutual consent of the physician and patient, the patient's dismissal of the physician, the services of the physician are no longer needed, or the physician properly withdraws from the physician/patient relationship."[30] Specific requirements for terminating a doctor-patient relationship vary among states, but they typically require reasonable notice provided by the physician in writing, and adequate time for the patient to identify another physician. Failure to terminate care properly may constitute patient abandonment and breach of physician duty if injury results, subjecting the provider to disciplinary action and potential civil liability.[30]

Legal and ethical guidelines govern the termination of care, but physicians are under no obligation to establish a doctor-patient relationship with a specific individual in ordinary circumstances. Providers could make their policy regarding vaccines clear to prospective patients at the time an initial appointment is scheduled. Those patients hesitant or opposed to vaccines would understand this policy and would be free to seek care elsewhere if so desired. Although this method reflects the importance of vaccination and the corresponding commitment of physicians using it, it is a missed opportunity for communication with patients or parents that might correct inaccurate perceptions and change attitudes in favor of vaccination. If patients hesitant about vaccines seek care only from so-called vaccine-friendly physicians open to any approach to vaccination, the debates and confusion surrounding vaccination are more likely to persist.

For patients in an established relationship with a physician, the AAP does not recommend terminating care in response to refusal of vaccines. A 2005 policy statement (renewed in 2010) states that continued refusal after discussion should be respected except in special cases such as outbreaks.[31] It adds:

> *However, when a substantial level of distrust develops, significant differences in the philosophy of care emerge, or poor quality of communication persists, the pediatrician may encourage the family to find another physician or practice...Such decisions should be unusual and generally made only after attempts have been made to work with the family. Families with doubts about immunization should still have access to good medical care, and maintaining the relationship in the face of*

disagreement conveys respect and at the same time allows the child access to medical care. Furthermore, a continuing relationship allows additional opportunity to discuss the issue of immunization over time.[31]

Continued communication with parents who refuse vaccines can produce favorable outcomes. A survey of parents who accepted vaccines after initially delaying or refusing them identified information obtained from health care providers as the most common reason for the change.[32]

The CDC takes a similar position against terminating treatment due to vaccine refusal. It recommends that instead of excluding patients who refuse vaccines, "an effective public health strategy is to identify common ground and discuss measures that need to be followed if the decision is to defer vaccination."[26]

Patients or parents refusing vaccines present a variety of challenges and potential frustrations for physicians who believe strongly in the benefits of vaccination, but the urge to respond with animosity or antagonism must be resisted. Beyond the legal and ethical complexities associated with terminating care, doing so as a general practice does nothing to advance the case for vaccination, forestalling the opportunity to subsequently change minds through continued education and dialog. It also may reinforce the divisions and distrust that explain the persistence of controversies over vaccine safety despite considerable evidence to the contrary.

Individuals with reservations about vaccines already believe that their voices are marginalized or ignored by the medical establishment. Rather than actions that would effectively establish parallel networks of care for parents and patients based on their views about vaccines, a far better solution is to continue open, honest, and factual communication about the risks and benefits of vaccines. These activities require ongoing dissemination of accurate information about vaccine safety and effectiveness, as well as support for continued research and surveillance to ensure that the considerable existing public trust in vaccination remains warranted.[33]

HEALTH CARE WORKER INFLUENZA VACCINATION

Discussions of vaccination refusal most often focus on parents hesitant about vaccines for their young children. While this group is the largest focus of vaccination programs and the most prominent source of controversies, reluctance to receive recommended vaccines is common among many populations. Increased attention in recent years has been directed toward the particular challenge of vaccination of health care workers against influenza.[34] Despite a long history of the prevention of influenza by means of vaccination and a recommendation since 1981 that health care workers receive the vaccine annually, obtaining satisfactory vaccination rates in this group has been notoriously difficult.[35]

Reasons provided by health care workers for why they choose not to receive influenza vaccination are particularly troubling, as they echo many of the inaccurate perceptions of the vaccine and the disease it prevents that are common among the public. These reasons include the false possibility of getting influenza from the vaccine, the allegedly mild nature of influenza, fear of needles, and an array of vaccine safety concerns unsupported by scientific evidence. Hospitals and other health care facilities have attempted a variety of strategies to boost vaccination rates, including incentives, active declination procedures, and appeals to professional duty. These strategies have all failed to produce adequate vaccination rates among health care workers.[35]

In 2004, the Virginia Mason Medical Center in Seattle became the first health care facility to mandate annual influenza vaccination as a condition of employment.[36]

The policy met resistance, particularly from unions representing some health care workers, but it proved remarkably effective at elevating vaccination rates to unprecedented levels. Dozens of health care facilities have adopted comparable policies in recent years, obtaining similarly favorable vaccination rates.[37]

Although requiring vaccination as a condition of employment is a significant action, the policy is justified by the obligations of physicians, nurses, and other health care professionals to protect the patients under their care and the clear failure of voluntary approaches. Some commentators have noted the unfortunate message that may be sent to the public about vaccines if health care providers must be compelled to receive them or risk losing their jobs.[38] Others note that having a fully vaccinated workforce sets an important example for the public. Allowing health care workers to remain unvaccinated places patients, including those highly susceptible to infections, at a greater risk of illness. This concern extends to hospitals as well as office settings. Health care workers are free to make personal health choices that place only themselves at increased risk of harm, but they may not endanger the health of the patients for whom they have a professional, ethical, and legal duty to protect. As the American Medical Association Code of Medical Ethics states, "A physician must recognize responsibility to patients first and foremost."[39]

SUMMARY

Resistance to vaccination is as old as vaccination itself.[40–42] Throughout this history, programs that have aimed to aggressively impose vaccination on an unwilling populace have largely failed, replaced by policies that educate and inform citizens while accepting that unanimity is a very difficult goal. Physicians, other health care providers, and the overall medical and public health communities should continue to unapologetically advocate for vaccination as one of the most valuable and successful tools for disease prevention. Health care professionals should carefully assess the safety and effectiveness of individual vaccines and the vaccination schedule, communicating clearly and accurately what is known and unknown about risks and benefits.

Health care providers should view individuals hesitant about or opposed to vaccines not as frustrations or threats to public health, but as opportunities to educate and inform. Excluding patients who question or oppose vaccines may appear to be an attractive method to demonstrate the importance of vaccination, but it leaves vulnerable infants and children without advocacy, and only adds to the climate of antagonism that often poisons contemporary discussions of vaccination in the United States. Through ongoing dialog, mutual respect for opposing views, and the demonstration of the importance of vaccination through one's own behavior, public support for vaccines can be preserved and broadened.

ACKNOWLEDGMENTS

The authors wish to thank Laura Backup for research assistance in the development of this article. They also wish to acknowledge the support of The Greenwall Foundation and the Center for Vaccine Ethics and Policy of the Children's Hospital of Philadelphia, The Wistar Institute, and the Center for Bioethics of the University of Pennsylvania.

REFERENCES

1. Wolfe RM, Sharp LK. Vaccination or immunization? The impact of search terms on the internet. MMWR Morb Mortal Wkly Rep 2005;10(6):537–51.

2. Godlee F, Smith J, Marcovitch H. Wakefield's article linking MMR vaccine and autism was fraudulent. BMJ 2011;342:c7452.
3. Committee on Infectious Diseases. Recommended childhood and adolescent immunization schedules—United States, 2011. Pediatrics 2011;127(2):387–8.
4. Offit PA, Quarles J, Gerber MA, et al. Addressing parents' concerns: do multiple vaccines overwhelm or weaken the infant's immune system? Pediatrics 2002;109: 124–9.
5. U.S. Court of Federal Claims. Omnibus autism proceeding. 2011. Available at: http://www.uscfc.uscourts.gov/omnibus-autism-proceeding. Accessed February 24, 2011.
6. Mnookin S. The panic virus: a true story of science, medicine, and fear. New York: Simon & Schuster; 2011.
7. Winter K, Harriman K, Schechter R, et al. Notes from the field: pertussis, California, January-June 2010. MMWR Morb Mortal Wkly Rep 2010;59(26):817.
8. Wooten KG, Kolasa M, Singleton JA, et al. National, state, and local area vaccination coverage among children ages 19-35 months—United States, 2009. MMWR Morb Mortal Wkly Rep 2010;59(36):1171–7.
9. Omer SB, Pan WK, Halsey NA, et al. Nonmedical exemptions to school immunization requirements: secular trends and association of state policies with pertussis incidence. JAMA 2006;296(14):1757–63.
10. Omer SB, Salmon D, Orenstein WA, et al. Vaccine refusal, mandatory immunization, and the risks of vaccine-preventable diseases. N Engl J Med 2009;360(19):1981–8.
11. Immunization Action Coalition. Available at: http://www.immunize.org/. Accessed February 27, 2011.
12. American Academy of Pediatrics. Immunization: just for pediatricians. Available at: http://www.aap.org/immunization/pediatricians/pediatricians.html. Accessed February 25, 2011.
13. Immunization Action Coalition. It's federal law: you must give your patients current vaccine information statements (VISs). Available at: http://www.immunize.org/catg.d/p2027.pdf. Accessed February 21, 2011.
14. Rosenthal SL, Weiss TW, Zimet GD, et al. Predictors of HPV vaccine uptake among women aged 19-26: importance of a physician's recommendation. Vaccine 2011; 29(5):890–5.
15. Sears R. The vaccine book: making the right decision for your child. New York: Little, Brown, and Company; 2007.
16. American Academy of Pediatrics. The childhood immunization schedule: why is it like that? Available at: http://www.aap.org/immunization/families/faq/Vaccineschedule.pdf. Accessed February 21, 2011.
17. Offit PA, Moser CA. The problem with Dr. Bob's alternate vaccine schedule. Pediatrics 2009;123(1):e164–9.
18. Nguyen HQ, Jumaan AO, Seward JF. Decline in mortality due to varicella after implementation of varicella vaccination in the United States. N Engl J Med 2005; 352:450–8.
19. Centers for Disease Control and Prevention. Parent's guide to childhood immunizations. Available at: http://www.cdc.gov/vaccines/pubs/parents-guide/downloads/parents-guide-part1.pdf. Accessed February 23, 2011.
20. American Academy of Pediatrics. Documenting parental refusal to have their children vaccinated. Available at: http://www.aap.org/immunization/pediatricians/pdf/RefusaltoVaccinate.pdf. Accessed February 26, 2011.
21. Flanagan-Klygis EA, Sharp L, Frader JE. Dismissing the family who refuses vaccines: a study of pediatrician attitudes. Arch Pediatr Adolesc Med 2005; 159:929–34.

22. Sears R. What is a vaccine-friendly doctor? Available at: AskDrSears.com; http://www.askdrsears.com/thevaccinebook/Vaccine_Friendly_Doctors.asp. Accessed February 25, 2011.
23. Orenstein WA, Rodewald LE, Hinman AR, et al. Immunization in the United States. In: Plotkin SA, Orenstein WA, Offit PA, editors. Vaccines. 5th edition. Philadelphia: Saunders; 2008. p. 1479–510.
24. Merck & Co., Inc. Merck Vaccine Patient Assistance Program. Available at: http://www.merck.com/merckhelps/vaccines/home.html. Accessed February 22, 2011.
25. GlaxoSmithKline. GSK Vaccine Access Program. Available at: http://www.gskforyou.com/18_programs.htm. Accessed February 22, 2011.
26. Kroger AT, Sumaya CV, Pickering LK, et al. General recommendations on vaccination: recommendations of the Advisory Committee on Immunization Practices (ACIP). MMWR Recomm Rep 2011;60(2):1–61.
27. American Academy of Pediatrics Committee on Bioethics. Informed consent, parental permission, and assent in pediatric practice. Pediatrics 1995;95(2):314–7.
28. Bonney LE, Lally M, Williams DR, et al. Where to begin human papillomavirus vaccination? Lancet Infect Dis 2006;6:389.
29. Offit B. Voices from the field: controversies in vaccine mandates. Curr Probl Pediatr Adolesc Health Care 2010;40:59–60.
30. Katz LL, Katz MB. When a physician may refuse to treat a patient. Physician's News Digest 2002;2.
31. Diekema DS, Committee on Bioethics. Responding to parental refusals of immunization of children. Pediatrics 2005;115(5):1428–31.
32. Gust DA, Darling N, Kennedy A, et al. Parents with doubts about vaccines: which vaccines and why? Pediatrics 2008;122(4):718–25.
33. Schwartz JL. Unintended consequences: the primacy of public trust in vaccination. Mich Law Rev First Impressions 2009;107:100–5.
34. Sullivan SJ, Jacobson RM, Poland GA. Mandating influenza vaccination for healthcare workers. Expert Rev Vaccines 2009;8(11):1469–74.
35. Poland GA, Tosh P, Jacobson RM. Requiring influenza vaccination for health care workers: seven truths we must accept. Vaccine 2005;23:2251–5.
36. Talbot TR, Schaffner W. On being the first: Virginia Mason Medical Center and mandatory influenza vaccination of healthcare workers. Infect Control Hosp Epidemiol 2010;31(9):889–92.
37. Feemster KA, Prasad P, Smith MJ, et al. Employee designation and health care worker support of an influenza vaccine mandate at a large pediatric tertiary care hospital. Vaccine 2011;29(9):1762–9.
38. Annas GJ. Don't force medical pros to get H1N1 vaccine. New York: Newsday, October 2, 2009.
39. American Medical Association. AMA code of medical ethics. Available at: http://www.ama-assn.org/ama/pub/physician-resources/medical-ethics/code-medical-ethics/principles-medical-ethics.shtml. Accessed March 4, 2011.
40. Durbach N. Bodily matters: the anti-vaccination movement in England, 1853–1907. Durham (NC): Duke University Press; 2005.
41. Colgrove J. State of immunity: the politics of vaccination in twentieth-century America. Berkeley (CA): University of California Press; 2006.
42. Offit PA. Deadly choices: how the anti-vaccine movement threatens us all. New York: Basic Books; 2010.

Office Immunization

Gary A. Emmett, MD[a,*], Melissa Schneider, MD, MSPH[b]

KEYWORDS

• Immunization • Vaccine • Diphtheria • Tetanus

Nothing has improved disease control as thoroughly as immunizations. In well-immunized populations, there is no flaccid paralysis (polio), almost no epiglottitis or postmeningitis deafness (*Haemophilus influenzae*), and little postviral male sterility (mumps). Immunizations are not perfect; they may cause side effects, some of which have led to the discontinuation of the vaccine when side effects have outweighed the vaccine's protective effects (eg, rotavirus vaccine and intussusception). However, immunization works best not by the protection it provides the individual but by the protection provided to the population at risk ("the herd effect"). Haemophilus influenzae type B (Hib) vaccine is a good example because it has no significant side effects that influence the final cost-effectiveness (cost-effectiveness considers all outcomes not just the monetary) of this immunization. A 2002 article in the United Kingdom cited a disease reduction of 97.4% when about 90% of children had received the full course of the vaccine. The immunogenicity of the conjugated Hib vaccines is close to 95%.[1] When about 40% of the population younger than 5 years was immunized in the United States with Hib vaccine, the disease rate had lowered by close to 75%, and, when 80% of the target population was immunized, the disease rate decreased by more than 90%. Thus, the herd effect protected a significant percentage of the unvaccinated susceptible population.[2]

Forces against vaccination have been vocal for well over 250 years. Many were against Jenner's smallpox vaccine, and it took 200 years to eliminate endemic smallpox from the earth. In the 1950s, there was great opposition to the oral polio vaccine in spite of the high frequency of death or disability from this endemic virus, including the visible disability of a president of the United States. Andrew Wakefield committed fraud in his study published in 1998 in the *Lancet* by creating false data linking measles-mumps-rubella (MMR) vaccine to autism and subsequently lost his license to practice medicine. Nonetheless, more than 20% of American parents believe that MMR vaccine and autism are directly connected, and a committed and vocal group of antivaccine activists has led to a high rate of MMR rejection by parents.

[a] Department of Pediatrics, Thomas Jefferson University, 833 Chestnut Street, Suite 300, Philadelphia, PA 19107, USA

[b] Grand Rapids Medical Education Partners, Helen DeVos Children's Hospital, 100 Michigan Street NE, Grand Rapids, MI 49503, USA

* Corresponding author.

E-mail address: gemmett@nemours.org

Prim Care Clin Office Pract 38 (2011) 729–745

doi:10.1016/j.pop.2011.07.010 **primarycare.theclinics.com**

0095-4543/11/$ – see front matter

According to a 2010 Centers for Disease Control and Prevention (CDC) report, 40% of American parents with young children have delayed or refused 1 or more vaccines for their child because of their fear of side effects. High rates of MMR rejection by parents has resulted in measles once again being endemic in England and Wales, killing children in Great Britain every year. What is clear is that there is no correlation between immunization and autism or other major developmental problems. However, any agent that may cause fever in young children, including viruses and bacteria, may cause seizures in susceptible individuals and, in rare incidents, result in developmental problems. Vaccination experts such as Offit[3] believe that the combination of relative rarity of serious infectious diseases in the developed world (because of immunizations) and the prevalence of minor fevers and illnesses in children, which may be temporally (and coincidentally) related to immunization, lead to high immunization rejection by parents. Parents do not realize the urgency of immunization for their children and fear that the immunizations themselves might hurt their children.

Several vaccine-related factors in the last 2 decades in the United States have improved the safety of children and compensated children with alleged adverse reactions to immunizations:

- The Vaccines for Children (VFC) program
  The VFC became operational on October 1, 1994. Known as section 1928 of the Social Security Act, the VFC program is an entitlement program (a right granted by law) for eligible children, aged 18 years and less. The VFC program helps families of children who may not otherwise have access to vaccines by providing free vaccines to doctors who serve them. Providers are not allowed to charge for these vaccines but may charge a minimal fee for administration of vaccines. The VFC is administered at the national level by the CDC, which contracts with vaccine manufacturers to buy vaccines at reduced rates. States and eligible projects enroll physicians who serve eligible patients up to and including age 18 years and who provide routine immunizations. Vaccines available from the VFC at the time this article is written include diphtheria/tetanus/pertussis, Hib, hepatitis A, hepatitis B, human papillomavirus, influenza, MMR, meningococcal, pneumococcal 13, polio, rotavirus, and varicella vaccines of various combinations and strengths. Records of distribution of the VFC vaccines and eligibility of the recipients to receive VFC vaccines must be precisely kept by practitioners who distribute these immunizations. Lack of accurate records can result in the practitioner being removed from the program, or, in egregious examples, large fines and potential criminal prosecution.
- Vaccine Adverse Event Reporting System (VAERS)
  The VAERS is a postmarketing safety surveillance program, collecting information about adverse events (possible side effects) that occur after the administration of vaccines licensed for use in the United States. This program is jointly sponsored by the CDC and the Food and Drug Administration. Providers are required to report adverse events of vaccines that come to their attention. If an unusual or serious reaction occurs, a form is available online (https://vaers.hhs.gov/esub/step1).
- National Vaccine Injury Compensation Program (VICP)
  On October 1, 1988, the National Childhood Vaccine Injury Act of 1986 created VICP, which is a no-fault resolution program for parents who think a vaccine has injured their child. This effort involves multiple government agencies, including

the Health Resources and Services Agency. They can be contacted at http://www.hrsa.gov/vaccinecompensation/default.htm.[4]

Immunization schedules are issued annually by the CDC. Below are listed relevant websites for the current schedules, which are also published in the *Mortality and Morbidity Weekly Report* issued weekly by the CDC:

http://www.cdc.gov/vaccines/recs/schedules/default.htm (CDC current vaccination schedules)[5]
http://www.cdc.gov/vaccines/recs/schedules/child-schedule.htm#printable (catch-up schedules for underimmunized children older than 4 months)[6]
http://www.cdc.gov/vaccines/pubs/ACIP-list.htm (CDC Advisory Committee on Immunization Practices [ACIP] recommendations)[7]
http://wwwnc.cdc.gov/travel/content/vaccinations.aspx (CDC traveler's health site with rules for administration and indications for use)[8]
http://www.immunize.org/vis (vaccine information sheets for each vaccine type)[9]
http://vaccinesafety.edu/package_inserts.htm (current package inserts for all vaccines)[10]

VACCINE ADMINISTRATION

Needle Selection (Right Equipment)

Age Group	Site	Length (in)	Gauge
Infants	Thigh	5/8–1	22–23
Older children	Thigh	7/8–1¼	22–25
	Deltoid	5/8–1¼	22–25
Adult men	Deltoid	1–1½	20–25
Women lighter than 70 kg	Deltoid	1	20–25
Women 70–100 kg	Deltoid	1¼	20–25
Women heavier than 100 kg, obese men	Deltoid	Perhaps 2	20–25

Proper Technique (Right Site and Right Administration Technique)

Subcutaneous (SC): pinch up skin, insert needle at a 45° to 90° angle so that its tip is inside the skin fold made by the pinch and inject. Pulling back first on the needle is no longer deemed necessary.

Intramuscular (IM): In children lighter than 10 kg and not ambulatory, use the anterolateral thigh. In older larger children and adults use the posterolateral upper arm. Grasp muscle; insert needle at 90° to the skin; pull back to see if the tip is in a blood vessel; and, if no blood flash, inject.

Time Out (Right Vaccine and Right Patient)

Many vaccines have similar names. DTaP (diphtheria and tetanus toxoids and acellular pertussis) and Tdap (tetanus toxoids and reduced diphtheria and acellular pertussis) vaccines are the most easily confused. Always have at least 2 people check vaccine orders (such as provider and nurse/technician) to prevent administrative errors. Check the name and birthday or at least one other personal information identifier before administration. Immunization may be administered inappropriately by using the wrong equipment, the wrong site, the wrong administration technique, the wrong vaccine, or the wrong patient.

CURRENTLY AVAILABLE VACCINES (AS OF FEBRUARY 1, 2011)

Anthrax

Trade Name	Constituents	Notes	Rules of Administration
BioThrax	Inactivated anthrax	• Not recommended for use in the general public. Should only be used after public health or infectious disease consultation • Recommended for preexposure prophylaxis for certain laboratory & military personnel or postexposure prophylaxis along with appropriate antimicrobials	• Approved for ages 18–65 y • 5 doses (0.5 mL IM) for those who may be exposed to large amounts of anthrax at d 0; wk 4; & mo 6, 12, & 18 followed by annual boosters • 3 doses (0.5 mL SC) for persons exposed to anthrax with first dose as soon after exposure as possible & the second & third doses 2 & 4 wk after the first dose plus appropriate antimicrobial therapy for 60 d

BCG (Tuberculosis)

Trade Name	Constituents	Notes	Rules of Administration
BCG Vaccine U.S.P.	Live attenuated *Mycobacterium bovis*	Rarely indicated in the US. Contact the TB control program in the area or the CDC's Division of Tuberculosis Elimination	Standard childhood shot in countries with active TB, such as India & China

Diphtheria and Tetanus (Tetanus and Diphtheria Toxoid, Diphtheria and Tetanus Toxoid, DTap, Tdap, and Combinations Vaccines)

All products are interchangeable as long as they are appropriate for the age of the patient.

Once primary series is completed, children (≤18 years of age) should receive a booster every 5 years and adults (≥19 years of age) should receive a booster every 10 years or if exposed to a potential tetanus contaminated wound and no booster in those time limits.

Trade Name	Constituents	Notes	Rules of Administration
DT (generic)	Diphtheria & tetanus toxoids	• For use when there is contraindication to the pertussis component of DTaP • Multidose vial contains thimerosal	• *Approved for ages 6 wk–6 y* • 5-dose series (0.5 mL IM) at ages 2, 4, 6, & 15–20 mo & 4–6 y
Decavac & Td (generic)	Diphtheria & tetanus toxoids	• Also given for wound prophylaxis with or without immune globulin	• *Approved for age ≥7 y* • As primary immunization, 3-dose (0.5 mL IM) series with first 2 doses 4–8 wk apart & third dose 6–12 mo after second dose • As booster, 1 dose (0.5 mL IM) every 10 y
Daptacel, Infanrix, & Tripedia (DTaP)[a]	Tetanus, diphtheria toxoids, & acellular pertussis	• Contraindicated in persons with a history of encephalopathy within 7 d of previous pertussis-containing vaccine without other identifiable cause or in persons with progressive neurologic disorders	• *All are approved for ages >6 wk & <7 y* • 5-dose (0.5 mL IM) series given at ages 2, 4, 6, & 15–20 mo & 4–6 y • Fourth dose may be given as early as 12 mo of age provided that 6 mo have elapsed since third dose
Boostrix & Adacel (Tdap)[a]	Tetanus, diphtheria toxoids, & acellular pertussis	• As above for DTaP	• *Boostrix, approved for ages 10–64 y* • *Adacel, approved for ages 11–64 y* • *The ACIP recommends use of Tdap in adults aged >65 y who have close contact with an infant <12 mo* • *Children aged 7–10 y who are not fully vaccinated against pertussis should receive a single dose of Tdap* • *As booster only, 1 dose (0.5 mL IM) once in lifetime*
TriHIBit[b]	DTaP/Hib	• As above for DTaP	• *Approved for ages 15–18 mo* who have received 3 previous doses of DTap & Hib • Used as the fourth dose only (0.5 mL IM) of both the DTap & Hib series • Tripedia is used to reconstitute ActHIB to make TriHIBit

(*continued on next page*)

Trade Name	Constituents	Notes	Rules of Administration
Kinrix[b]	DTaP/IPV	• As above for DTaP	• *Approved for ages 4–6 y* • Used as the fifth dose (0.5 mL IM) of DTaP series & fourth dose of IPV series in those whose first 3 DTaP doses have been Infanrix/Pediarix & whose fourth dose was Infanrix
Pentacel[b]	DTaP/IPV/Hib	• As above for DTaP	• *Approved for ages 6 wk–4 y* • 4-dose series (0.5 mL IM) at ages 2, 4, 6, & 15–18 mo
Pediarix[b]	DTaP/HepB/IPV	• As above for DTaP	• *Approved for ages 6 wk–6 y* • 3-dose series (0.5 mL IM) at ages 2, 4, & 6 mo

Abbreviations: DT, tetanus and diphtheria toxoid; HepB, hepatitis B; IPV, inactivated polio vaccine; Td, diphtheria and tetanus toxoid.

[a] See differences in italics.

[b] Combination vaccine.

Hib

Trade Name	Constituents	Notes	Rules of Administration
PedvaxHIB, ActHIB, HibTITER, & Hiberix[a]	Inactivated conjugate Hib	—	• ActHIB, *approved for ages 2–18 mo in infants aged 7–11 mo receiving a 2-dose (0.5 mL IM) series at 8-wk intervals & a booster at ages 15–18 mo & in children aged >12 mo receiving 1 dose (0.5 mL IM) followed by a booster 2 mo later* • PedvaxHIB & HibTITER, *approved for ages 2–71 mo for infants aged 2–11 mo receiving a 2-dose (0.5 mL IM) series 2 mo apart & children aged >15 mo receiving 1 dose (0.5 mL IM), all followed by a booster at 15 mo but not less than 2 mo after previous dose* • Hiberix, *approved for ages 15 mo–4 y as 1 booster (0.5 mL IM) dose for children completing a 2-dose series before age 12 mo*

(continued on next page)

Trade Name	Constituents	Notes	Rules of Administration
Comvax[a]	Inactivated Hib/HepB	• Contraindicated in persons with a history of hypersensitivity or life-threatening reaction to yeast	• *Approved for ages 6wk to 15 mo born of HepB-negative mothers*[a] • *3-dose (0.5 mL IM) series at ages 2, 4, & 12–15 mo*[a]
TriHIBit[b]	DTaP/Hib	• See "Diphtheria and Tetanus"	• See "Diphtheria and Tetanus"
Pentacel[b]	DTaP/IPV/Hib	• See "Diphtheria and Tetanus"	• See "Diphtheria and Tetanus"

Abbreviations: HepB, hepatitis B; IPV, inactivated polio vaccine.
[a] See differences in italics.
[b] Combination vaccine.

Hepatitis A

Trade Name	Constituents	Notes	Rules of Administration
Havrix & Vaqta[a]	Inactivated HepA virus	• Approved for ages ≥1 y	• For children aged 12 mo–18 y, 2 doses of (0.5 mL IM) at least 6 mo apart • Optimal administration of second dose, *6–12 mo (Havrix)/6–18 mo (Vaqta)* after first dose • For adults aged ≥19 y, 2 doses (1 mL IM) at the same above schedule
Twinrix[b]	Inactivated HepA/HepB	• Contraindicated in persons with a history of hypersensitivity or life-threatening reaction to yeast & neomycin	• *Approved for ages ≥18 y* • 3 doses (1 mL IM) at 0, 1, & 6 mo or 4-dose schedule on days 0, 7, & 21–30 followed by a booster dose at 12 mo

Abbreviations: HepA, hepatitis A; HepB, hepatitis B.
[a] See differences in italics.
[b] Combination vaccine.

Hepatitis B

Trade Name	Constituents	Notes	Rules of Administration
Engerix-B & Recombivax HB[a]	Inactivated HepB virus	• Contraindicated in persons with a history of hypersensitivity or life-threatening reaction to yeast • Pregnant women who need protection from HepB infection may be vaccinated • For babies born to mothers who are HepB surface antigen positive, vaccine must be administered within 12 h of birth & immune globulin (HBiG) (0.5 mL IM) should be given within 7 d of birth. Baby must receive second HepB vaccine 28–35 d later for maximum protection	• For children, 3-dose (0.5 mL IM) series; first dose at birth, second dose 1 mo after first dose, & third dose at least 2 mo after second dose & at least 4 mo after the first dose. Must be ≥6 mo of age for third dose. • For adults, 3-dose (1 mL IM) series; second dose 1 mo after first dose & third dose at least 2 mo after second dose & at least 4 mo after the first dose • For adults receiving hemodialysis or with other immuno-compromising conditions: ○ *Engerix-B, 2 doses (1 mL IM) of 20 μg/mL administered simultaneously at separate sites on a 4-dose schedule at 0, 1, 2, & 6 mo* ○ *Recombivax HB, 1 dose (1 mL IM) of 40 μg/mL on the above 3-dose adult schedule*
Twinrix[b]	Inactivated HepA/HepB	• See "Hepatitis A"	• See "Hepatitis A"
Comvax[b]	Inactivated Hib/HepB	• See "Hib"	• See "Hib"
Pediarix[b]	DTaP/HepB/IPV	• See "Diphtheria & Tetanus"	• See "Diphtheria & Tetanus"

Abbreviations: HepA, hepatitis A; HepB, hepatitis B; IPV, inactivated polio vaccine.

[a] See differences in italics.

[b] Combination vaccine.

Human Papillomavirus

Trade Name	Constituents	Notes	Rules of Administration
Gardasil & Cervarix[a]	Inactivated HPV types 6, 11, 16, 18 & (Gardasil); inactivated HPV types 16 & 18 (Cervarix)	• It is not recommended for pregnant women, but receiving the vaccine when pregnant is not a reason to consider termination of the pregnancy	• Gardasil, approved for use in female *& male* populations aged 9–26 y • Cervarix, approved for use in girls and women aged 9–26 y • 3-dose schedule (0.5 mL IM) with second dose 1–2 mo after first dose & third dose 6 mo after first dose • Administration to patients aged ≥27 y is under consideration by the FDA & CDC at the time of publication • Men may receive the Gardasil vaccine, but it is not required or formally recommended[11]

Abbreviation: HPV, human papillomavirus.
[a] See differences in italics.

Influenza (Flu)

Trade Name	Constituents	Notes	Rules of Administration
Afluria, Fluzone, Fluzone High-Dose, Fluarix, Fluvirin, FluLaval & Agriflu[a]	*Inactivated* trivalent flu	• Contraindicated in persons with a history of hypersensitivity or life-threatening reaction to egg • FluLaval, Afluria (multidose vial), Fluvirin (multidose vial), & Fluzone (multidose vial) contain thimerosal	• Afluria & Fluzone, *approved for ages ≥6 mo* • Fluarix, *approved for ages ≥3 y* • Fluvirin, *approved for ages ≥4 y* • Agriflu & FluLaval, *approved for ages ≥18 y* • Fluzone High-Dose, *approved for ages ≥65 y* • Recommended yearly vaccination • 6 mo–35 mo of age, 1 dose (*0.25 mL IM*) for previously vaccinated (for flu) & 2 doses for previously unvaccinated 1 mo apart • 36 mo–8 y of age, 1 dose (*0.5 mL IM*) for previously vaccinated & 2 doses for previously unvaccinated 1 mo apart • ≥9 y of age, 1 dose (*0.5 mL IM*)

(*continued on next page*)

Trade Name	Constituents	Notes	Rules of Administration
FluMist[a]	*Live* attenuated trivalent flu	• Contraindicated in persons with a history of hypersensitivity or life-threatening reaction to eggs, gelatin, gentamicin, or arginine or with primary or acquired immunodeficiency • Contraindicated in concomitant aspirin therapy in children & adolescents • Do not use in persons with recent history of asthma	• *Approved for 2–49 y of age* • 24 mo–8 y of age, 1 dose (0.2 mL; *0.1 mL per nostril*) for previously vaccinated & 2 doses for previously unvaccinated 1 mo apart • 9–49 y of age, 1 dose (*0.2 mL, 0.1 mL in each nostril*)

[a] See differences in italics.

Japanese Encephalitis

Trade Name	Constituents	Notes	Rules of Administration
JE-VAX[a]	Inactivated JE (Mouse brain derived)	• Indicated for travel to countries with active JE such as rural areas of Japan. See CDC indications for use • Contains thimerosal	• *Approved for ages ≥1 y* • *3 doses* (1 mL SC) for persons aged ≥3 y at 0, 7, & 30 d • *3 doses (0.5 mL SC)* for children of 1 & 2 y of age at 0, 7, & 30 d
Ixiaro[a]	Inactivated JE (Vero cell culture derived)	—	• *Approved for ages ≥17 y* • *2 doses (0.5 mL IM)* at 0 & 28 d

Abbreviation: JE, Japanese encephalitis.
[a] See differences in italics.

MMR

Trade Name	Constituents	Notes	Rules of Administration
Attenuvax, Mumpsvax, & Meruvax	Live attenuated measles (Attenuvax), mumps (Mumpsvax), & rubella (Meruvax)	• No longer in production as of September 2010	—

(*continued on next page*)

Trade Name	Constituents	Notes	Rules of Administration
M-M-R II[a]	Live attenuated measles, mumps, & rubella viruses	• Contraindicated in persons with primary or acquired immunodeficiency & pregnant women	• *Approved for ages 12 mo* • 1 dose (0.5 mL SC) at 12–15 mo of age & 1 booster dose (0.5 mL SC) at 4–6 y of age
ProQuad[a]	MMR/varicella	• As above for M-M-R II • Use caution in persons with hypersensitivity to eggs or neomycin • **The AAP recommends that this vaccine only be used in children aged ≥4 y**	• *Approved for ages 12 mo–12 y* • Dosing schedule as above

Abbreviation: AAP, American Academy of Pediatrics.
[a] See differences in italics.

Meningococcal

Trade Name	Constituents	Notes	Rules of Administration
Menomune	Tetravalent meningococcal polysaccharide	• Menomune is an acceptable alternative if the conjugate versions are unavailable • Multidose vial contains thimerosal	• *Approved for ages 2–55 y* • 1 dose (0.5 mL *SC*) • Revaccination may be necessary with conjugate version, especially if vaccinated at age <4 y
Menactra & Menveo[a]	Tetravalent meningococcal conjugate	• Conjugate vaccine is preferred over polysaccharide in persons aged 11–55 y	• Recommended at ages 11–19 & 2–55 y in persons at increased risk • *Menactra, approved for ages 2–55 y* • *Menveo, approved for ages 11–55 y* • 1 dose (0.5 mL *IM*) after eleventh birthday, a second dose after sixteenth birthday is recommended before college

[a] See differences in italics.

Pneumococcal

Trade Name	Constituents	Notes	Rules of Administration
Prevnar13[a]	13-valent (Prevnar13) pneumococcal conjugate	• 7-valent (Prevnar) no longer in production as of 2010 • Children aged <16 mo who have only received Prevnar should get a Prevnar13 as soon as possible	• Prevnar, *approved for ages 6 wk–9 y* • Prevnar13, *approved for 6 wk–5 y* • 4 dose (0.5 mL *IM*) series at 2, 4, 6, & 12–15 mo
Pneumovax23	23-valent pneumococcal polysaccharide	—	• *Approved for ages 2 y* • Recommended routine vaccination at ages ≥65 y, in people with asthma/cigarette smokers aged 19–64 y, & in children aged ≥2 y with certain chronic conditions (ie, asplenism) • 1 dose (0.5 mL *SC or IM*). Booster may be given >5 y later if first dose was at age <64 y

[a] See differences in italics.

Polio

Trade Name	Constituents	Notes	Rules of Administration
Ipol	Inactivated poliovirus, 3 types (Mahoney, MEF-1, & Saukett)	• Contraindicated in persons with a history of hypersensitivity or life-threatening reaction to streptomycin, polymyxin B, & neomycin • Vaccination of pregnant women should be avoided	• 4 doses (0.5 mL SC) at ages 2, 4, & 6–18 mo & 4–6 y • Fourth dose is not necessary if the third dose was received on or after the fourth birthday • For adults & children who have missed primary series, first 2 doses should be administered at an interval of 4–8 wk & third dose should be administered 6–12 mo after second dose
Kinrix[a]	DTaP/IPV	• See "Diphtheria and Tetanus"	• See "Diphtheria and Tetanus"
Pentacel[a]	DTaP/IPV/Hib	• See "Diphtheria and Tetanus"	• See "Diphtheria and Tetanus"
Pediarix[a]	DTaP/HepB/IPV	• See "Diphtheria and Tetanus"	• See "Diphtheria and Tetanus"

Abbreviation: IPV, inactivated polio vaccine.
[a] Combination vaccine.

Rabies

Trade Name	Constituents	Notes	Rules of Administration
ImovaxRabies & RabAvert	Inactivated rabies virus	• Preexposure prophylaxis indicated for veterinarians, animal handlers, rabies researchers, and certain laboratory workers • Once initiated, rabies prophylaxis should not be interrupted or discontinued because of local or mild systemic adverse reactions • Immunosuppressive agents should not be administered during vaccination unless essential for treatment of other illnesses • The gluteal area should never be used as a vaccine injection area	• Postexposure prophylaxis, 5 doses (1 mL IM) at days 0, 3, 7, 14, & 28 plus immune globulin (20 IU/kg or 0.133 mL/kg of body weight) • Preexposure prophylaxis, 3 doses (1 mL IM) at days 0, 7 & 21, or 28 with serum antibody titer every 6 mo. Booster 1 dose if low titer

Rotavirus

Trade Name	Constituents	Notes	Rules of Administration
Rota Teq[a]	Live, attenuated, *pentavalent* human-bovine	• Caution should be used in the immunocompromised • The practitioner should not readminister a dose to an infant who regurgitates, spits out, or vomits during or after administration of the vaccine	• Minimum age for first dose is 6 wk • Maximum age for first dose is 14 wk and 6 d • Minimum interval between doses is 4 wk • Maximum age for last dose is 32 wk • *3-dose schedule with doses (2 mL po) at ages 2, 4, & 6 mo*
Rotarix[a]	Live, attenuated, *monovalent* human strain	• As above	• Minimum age for first dose is 6 wk • Maximum age for first dose is 14 wk and 6 d • Minimum interval between doses is 4 wk • Maximum age for last dose is 24 wk • *2-dose schedule with doses (1 mL po) at ages 2 & 4 mo*

[a] See differences in italics.

Smallpox

Trade Name	Constituents	Notes	Rules of Administration
Dryvax & ACAM2000	Live attenuated vaccinia virus	• Not commercially available • Available from the CDC for select laboratory, health care, & military personnel only	—

Typhoid

Trade Name	Constituents	Notes	Rules of Administration
Typhoid vaccine[a]	Parenteral heat/ phenol-inactivated vaccine	• Indicated for travel to countries with active typhoid. See CDC indications for use	• *Approved for ages ≥6 mo* • For ages 6 mo–10 y, *2 doses (0.25 mL SC)* at least 4 wk apart with a *booster every 3 y* • For ages ≥10 y, *2 doses (0.50 mL SC)* at least 4 wk apart with a *booster every 3 y* • *An intradermal formulation (0.10 mL) is available as a booster only, given every 3 y for ages ≥6 mo*
Typhim[a]	Capsular polysaccharide vaccine	• As above	• *Approved for ages ≥2 y* • *1 dose (0.50 mL IM)* • *Booster every 2 y*
Vivotif Berna[a]	*Live* attenuated Ty21a strain	• As above • Contraindicated in persons with primary or acquired immunodeficiency • Should not be given within 24 h of use of antimicrobials • Oral vaccine preferred over others when not contraindicated	• *Approved for ages ≥6 y* • *4-dose schedule, 1 dose (1 capsule po)* every 2 d • *Booster every 5 y* of the 4-dose schedule as above

[a] See differences in italics.

Varicella

Trade Name	Constituents	Notes	Rules of Administration
Varivax	Live attenuated varicella virus	• Contraindicated in persons with primary or acquired immunodeficiency & malignant neoplasms	• Approved for ages ≥1 y • For children aged ≤12 y, 2 doses (0.5 mL SC) at least 3 mo apart & recommended at ages 4–6 y • For adolescents and adults aged ≥13 y, 2 doses (0.5 mL SC) at least 4 wk apart
ProQuad[a]	MMR/varicella	• See "MMR"	—
Zostavax	Live attenuated herpes zoster	• See "Zoster"	—

[a] Combination vaccine.

Yellow Fever

Trade Name	Constituents	Notes	Rules of Administration
YF-Vax	Live attenuated 17D-204 virus strain	• Contraindicated in persons with a history of hypersensitivity or life-threatening reaction to eggs, chicken, & gelatin or in persons with primary or acquired immunodeficiency, malignant neoplasms, & transplants • For international travel, the vaccine must be administered by an approved vaccination center, & all vaccinees must possess a completed International Certificate of Vaccination or Prophylaxis, validated with provider's signature & official stamp. It is valid starting 10 d after vaccination & is good for 10 y	• Approved for ages ≥9 mo • 1 dose (0.5 mL SC) • Booster given at 10-y intervals

Zoster

Trade Name	Constituents	Notes	Rules of Administration
Zostavax	Live attenuated herpes zoster	• Contraindicated in persons with a history of hypersensitivity or life-threatening reaction to gelatin & neomycin or in persons with primary or acquired immunodeficiency • It should not be administered to persons of any age who have received the varicella vaccine • Persons with a reported history of zoster can receive the vaccine	• Licensed for ages ≥60 y • 1 dose (0.65 mL SC)

Notes: All vaccines are contraindicated in persons with a history of hypersensitivity or life-threatening reaction to any component of the vaccine with the exception of the rabies vaccine.

ACKNOWLEDGMENTS

We would like to acknowledge the massive amount of time contributed by Megan Lundy, Stephanie Bernard, and Lauren Daley in gathering information, developing the format, and fact checking all the information.

REFERENCES

1. Heath PT, McVernon J. The UK HIB vaccine experience. Arch Dis Child 2002;86:396–9.
2. Adegbola RA, Secka O, Lahai G, et al. Elimination of Haemophilus influenzae type b (Hib) disease from The Gambia after the introduction of routine immunisation with a Hib conjugate vaccine: a prospective study. Lancet 2005;366(9480):144–50.
3. Offit PA. Deadly choices: how the anti-vaccine movement threatens us all. New York (NY): Basic Books; 2011.
4. Health Resources and Services Administration. National Vaccine Injury Compensation Program. Available at: http://www.hrsa.gov/vaccinecompensation/default.htm. Accessed August 19, 2011.
5. Centers for Disease Control and Prevention. Vaccines & immunizations: immunization schedules. Available at: http://www.cdc.gov/vaccines/recs/schedules/default.htm. Accessed August 19, 2011.
6. Centers for Disease Control and Prevention. Vaccines & immunizations: 2011 child & adolescent immunization schedules. Available at: http://www.cdc.gov/vaccines/recs/schedules/child-schedule.htm#printable. Accessed August 19, 2011.

7. Centers for Disease Control and Prevention. Advisory Committee for Immunization Practices Recommendations. Available at: http://www.cdc.gov/vaccines/pubs/ACIP-list.htm. Accessed August 19, 2011.
8. Centers for Disease Control and Prevention. Travelers' health: vaccinations. Available at: http://wwwnc.cdc.gov/travel/content/vaccinations.aspx. Accessed August 19, 2011.
9. Immunization action coalition. Vaccination information for healthcare professionals. Available at: http://www.immunize.org/vis. Accessed August 19, 2011.
10. Institute for Vaccine Safety, Johns Hopkins Bloomberg School of Public Health. Package inserts and manufacturers for some US licensed vaccines and immunoglobulins. Available at: http://vaccinesafety.edu/package_inserts.htm. Accessed August 19, 2011.
11. Giuliano AR, Palefsky JM, Goldstone S, et al. Efficacy of quadrivalent HPV vaccine against HPV infection and disease in males. N Engl J Med 2011;364(5):401–11.

Keeping Up-to-Date with Immunization Practices

Donald B. Middleton, MD[a,*], Richard K. Zimmerman, MD, MPH[a], Judith A. Troy[a], Robert M. Wolfe, MD[b]

KEYWORDS

• Immunization • Vaccination • Shots • Vaccines • ACIP • STFM

In toto, immunizations constitute one of the most significant effective scientific advances in history.[1,2] All preventive health care workers should command a general knowledge of immunization basics, including available vaccines, routine vaccination schedules, common side effects, and routes of administration. The Advisory Council on Immunization Practices (ACIP) annually updates the unified vaccine schedules, which the American Academy of Family Practice (AAFP), the American Academy of Pediatrics (AAP), and the American College of Physicians (ACP) all endorse, and publishes the new schedules usually in January or February. In between these updates, established vaccines may gain new indications, may be provided in new combination, may have new precautions, or are found to work less well than initially hoped and new vaccines may become available. Outbreaks of vaccine-preventable disease (VPD) often alter vaccine recommendations.

Current vaccine schedules call for routine vaccination against 17 VPDs. Universal vaccination is extremely successful. Diseases such as polio are potentially conquerable worldwide. Others, including anthrax, cholera, rabies, yellow fever, and typhoid fever, are controllable. The 2010 outbreak of cholera in Haiti points to the need to continue to develop effective vaccines for potentially disastrous illnesses. New vaccine strategies are under development for universal influenza vaccine, and new

---

Disclosure: Current advisory committee on vaccination for Merck & Co, Inc; previous advisory committees on vaccination for Sanofi Pasteur, Pfizer, and GlaxoSmithKline (D.B.M.). Research grants from Merck, Sanofi Pasteur, and Medimmune and consultant to MedImmune (R.K.Z.). Speakers bureau for Merck and Sanofi Pasteur, consultant for both companies, and research grant from Sanofi Pasteur (R.M.W.). None (J.A.T.).

[a] Department of Family Medicine, University of Pittsburgh School of Medicine, 3518 Fifth Avenue, Pittsburgh, PA 15261, USA

[b] Department of Family Medicine, Pritzker School of Medicine, University of Chicago and NorthShore University HealthSystem, 6810 North McCormick Boulevard, Lincolnwood, IL 60712-2709, USA

* Corresponding author. UPMC St Margaret, 815 Freeport Road, Pittsburgh, PA 15215.
E-mail address: middletondb@upmc.edu

Prim Care Clin Office Pract 38 (2011) 747–761
doi:10.1016/j.pop.2011.07.011 primarycare.theclinics.com
0095-4543/11/$ – see front matter

routes of administration, such as the newly Food and Drug Administration (FDA)-approved intradermal injection route for influenza vaccine, are close to fruition.

A new vaccine takes time to develop. After assessing disease burden, researchers must develop an effective epitope, determine an appropriate antigen dose, and establish vaccine efficacy and safety.

The new vaccine must then receive FDA approval, after which the ACIP offers advice as to how to use it in a cost-effective manner and, if appropriate, list it on the routine schedules. Some new vaccines establish effectiveness through demonstration of disease prevention, but, because of the rarity of these clinical illnesses, most vaccines must only prove to induce antibody levels that are not inferior to those produced by currently available vaccines. Vaccine-induced antibody levels generally must be higher than the correlate of protection for a particular illness, that is, the antibody level that is known to prevent clinical disease. The new vaccine can then be incorporated into the ACIP schedule. Older products may be combined into new combinations to reduce administration and storage costs and multiple vaccinations at one visit, while simultaneously enhancing timely compliance with the vaccine schedules. An example of this process is the current recommendation to use Kinrix (diphtheria and tetanus toxoids and acellular pertussis/inactivated polio vaccine combination) at the booster dose for children aged 4 to 6 years. Kinrix was not shown to prevent tetanus, but it was shown to produce antibody levels that were noninferior to prior vaccine products and were above the correlate of protection antibody level for tetanus, and it saves one injection.[3]

Practitioners of preventive health should stay on schedule with vaccine recommendations as closely as possible. The reasons for doing so include primary prevention of VPDs, reducing outbreaks, and financial issues that include rewards for staying on target with 2011 Healthcare Effectiveness Data and Information Set goals. Many insurers financially reward practices for keeping their patients up-to-date. Healthy People 2020 (http://www.healthypeople.gov/2020) sets extremely high goals for vaccination of adults, despite the failure to meet Healthy People 2010 goals (**Fig. 1**). Besides changes in vaccination schedules, barriers to keeping current include the time required to do so, vaccine management and storage, incorporation of new immunization advice into practice, financial issues including vaccine cost and payment, and separation of Vaccines for Children (VFC) products from private supplies. Patient, parent, or physician reluctance to use some vaccines acts as a major barrier to keeping current. As VPDs become infrequent, the importance of vaccine side effects escalates. Every effort should be made to keep each patient on target with vaccinations. Sources to combat antivaccine sentiments include Web sites from the Centers for Disease Control and Prevention (CDC), AAP, and AAFP and numerous publications such as Dr Paul Offit's book, DeadlyChoices, published in 2011.[4]

This article is devoted to helping those in primary care to stay current with vaccine advice. In view of the many available sources for vaccine information, we have emphasized our primary choices to stay current but recognize that many other sources provide valuable information. Staying current with travel recommendations is difficult for even the most knowledgeable physician. This article provides some insight into the resources available to achieve this task as well.

ELECTRONIC HEALTH RECORDS AND IMMUNIZATION REGISTRIES

Immunization information systems (IIS), or immunization registries, are confidential, population-based, computerized databases that record all immunization doses administered by participating providers to persons residing within a given geopolitical

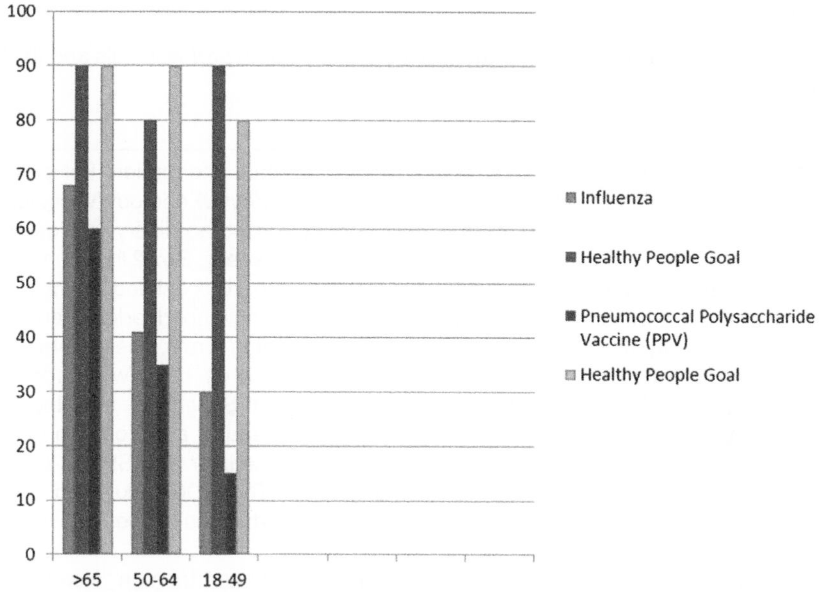

Fig. 1. Healthy People 2020 goals versus 2008 actual vaccination rates for influenza and pneumococcal vaccines. (*Data from* US Department of Health and Human Services. Healthy People 2020. Available at: http://www.healthypeople.gov/2020/topicsobjective2020. Accessed August 28, 2011.)

area.[5] One of the national health objectives for 2020 is to increase to 95% the proportion of children aged 6 years or less who participate in fully operational population-based IIS.[6] Overall in the United States, approximately 77% of children aged 6 years or less (18.4 million) participated in an IIS in 2009.[7]

Most practices have or plan to incorporate an electronic health record (EHR) system, which should be the ideal source of immunization information and support for clinical providers. Linkage to centralized information systems could both store the patient's immunization information and assess the patient's immunization needs. Ideally, EHR programmers should update the internal vaccination schedule so that the practitioner receives timely reminders to stay current for every patient visit. At present, numerous barriers, including development of standards for communication between EHRs and registries and clarification of rules regulating the exchange of protected health information between states, stand in the way of reaching this goal.[8] Of course, EHR vaccine information must also be regularly updated. The astute provider may be aware of vaccine changes before EHR update and, if a conduit is open to discussion with programmers, make a timely contribution to keeping vaccine recommendations current.

The American Recovery and Reinvestment Act (ARRA) of 2009 provides $19.2 billion of funding for health information technology (IT) to promote the use of EHRs. Title XIII of ARRA, Health Information Technology for Economic and Clinical Health Act (HITECH), enumerates provisions intended to accelerate adoption of certified EHR systems, standardization of EHR products, growth in the health IT workforce, and exchange of secure health data between partners.[6] A key part of HITECH is the EHR Incentive Program, administered by the Centers for Medicare and Medicaid Services, which requires physicians seeking full reimbursement to adopt EHRs that can transmit health information to immunization registries, a national priority.[9]

WEB SITES

Most of the listed Web sites have materials intended for both professionals and the lay public.

CDC

Box 1 lists federal and state immunization program contact information. For general immunization information, the CDC information at http://www.cdc.gov/vaccines is unparalleled (**Fig. 2**). The amount of information available is extraordinary, but knowing how to navigate the CDC site is critical to finding what one seeks. **Box 2** lists numerous topics for detailed review. The site also provides updates in a box entitled "In the Spotlight." Clicking on "Immunization Schedules" leads to the childhood, adolescent, and adult schedules (**Fig. 3**) and vaccine recording and screening forms. The general CDC immunization schedules page for health professionals is at http://www.cdc.gov/vaccines/recs/schedules/default.htm. Clicking on "Adult Schedule" and then on "Health Care Professionals" and scrolling down to "Schedules and Tools to Download" lead to 2 useful items: the adult immunization scheduler and Shots 2011 by the Society of Teachers of Family Medicine (STFM). The CDC's flu Web site is www.cdc.gov/flu. The CDC also offers educational opportunities online, via webinar, or for self-study.

Clicking on either the childhood or adolescent schedule and then on "Health Care Professionals" and scrolling down lead to the catch-up schedule. The catch-up schedule contains an interactive catch-up scheduler, a downloadable tool. Both the interactive childhood and adolescent catch-up scheduler and the adult immunization scheduler are regularly updated and serve as excellent means to staying current with a particular patient. Unfortunately, they do take a bit of time to use. Interested parents and patients can use these tools on their own once they are made aware of their location.

The CDC also offers an automatic notification of new information. The interested practitioner can sign up for this e-mail help at www.cdc.gov/emailupdates/index.html. A small box entitled "Get Email Updates" is also present at the www.cdc.gov/ Web site (see **Fig. 2**). Scrolling down in this same column leads to vaccines for travelers, providing information about vaccines required based on the destination. The direct link is http://wwwnc.cdc.gov/travel/content/vaccinations.aspx.

Vaccine information statements (VISs), extremely important to document that individuals were informed about vaccine indications and risks, are on the lower left-hand

Box 1
Federal and state immunization program contacts at http://www.cdc.gov/vaccines/news/newsltrs/imwrks/default.htm

E-mail immunization questions to NIPINFO@cdc.gov

State immunization program managers: http://www2a.cdc.gov/nip/progmgr/fieldstaff.asp?rpt=pm

VFC program, including state VFC program managers: http://www.cdc.gov/vaccines/programs/vfc/default.htm

IISs (immunization registries), including state IIS program managers: http://www.cdc.gov/vaccines/programs/iis/default.htm

Portal to all immunization programs such as VFC and state immunization departments: http://www.cdc.gov/vaccines/programs/default.htm

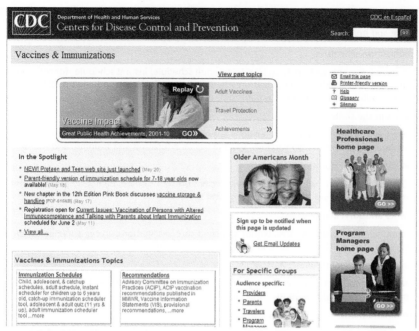

Fig. 2. CDC Vaccines & Immunization. (*Data from* Available at: http://www.cdc.gov/vaccines/. Accessed August 28, 2011.)

side. Some practitioners have dismissed patients who have refused vaccinations. The AAP does not advise automatic dismissal but rather encourages education. Whether education will be effective in increasing vaccination rates is unclear.

Some experts advise that parents who refuse vaccinations for their children sign the VIS, kept in the patient's chart. This approach documents that immunizations were refused by the parent or patient.

The Comprehensive Clinic Assessment Software Application, an immunization assessment tool for assessing immunization practices within a clinic, private practice, or any other environment where immunization is provided, presented under CDC auspices, is at http://www.cdc.gov/vaccines/programs/cocasa/default.htm, and the Assessment, Feedback, Incentives, and Exchange program to improve vaccination rates is at http://www.cdc.gov/vaccines/programs/afix/default.htm.

ACIP

Clicking on the CDC home page immunization schedules leads to the vaccines and immunization page. The right-hand column contains a link to ACIP recommendations (http://www.cdc.gov/vaccines/recs/acip), published shortly after each ACIP meeting, which typically occurs 3 times a year. Scrolling down on the ACIP recommendations site leads to vaccine-specific recommendations. As ACIP recommendations are published, the advice regarding a particular vaccine is updated in this Web site, making it an extremely useful site to update insurers and EHRs about recommended use of vaccinations.

Other Web Sites

Immunization action coalition

A nonprofit organization, the unparalleled Immunization Action Coalition (IAC) Web site (www.immunize.org/) has a wealth of easy-to-access informational materials,

Box 2
Vaccine and immunization topics

Immunization schedules

Child, adolescent, and catch-up schedules; adult schedule; instant scheduler for children up to 6 years old; catch-up immunization scheduler tool; adolescent and adult quiz (ages $\geq$11 years); adult immunization scheduler tool; and more

Vaccines in the United States

Vaccine shortages and delays questions answered about vaccines, who should not be vaccinated, potential new vaccines, vaccine basics, education and training, and more

Basic and common questions

Common questions, why immune, how vaccines prevent disease, immunity types, common misconceptions, risks of not vaccinating, and more

Statistics and surveillance

Immunization coverage rates, school and child care vaccination surveys, surveillance Web sites, related articles, manual and worksheets, and more

Education and training

Net conferences on current issues, podcasts, courses and materials, patient education materials, "You call the Shots," and more

Recommendations

The ACIP vaccination recommendations published in *Morbidity and Mortality Weekly Report*, vaccine information statements (VIS), provisional recommendations, and more

Vaccines and preventable diseases

What diseases are vaccine preventable, questions answered, about specific diseases, photo of diseases, and more

Vaccine side effects and safety

Possible vaccine side effects, concerns about the safety of vaccines, vaccine safety research, vaccine safety data link project, report a vaccine adverse reaction, and more

Requirements and laws

School requirement, state requirements, exemptions and consent forms, VIS, and more

Partners

Partners' Web sites, immunization-related Web sites, state and local health departments, related government agencies, and more

Data from the CDC Web site home page. Available at: http://cdc.gov/vaccines/. Accessed August 28, 2011.

including VISs in multiple languages and videos of numerous immunization issues. The site contains excellent summary tables and questionnaires for child, teenager, and adult immunizations. An additional IAC Web site, www.vaccineinformation.org/, is designed for both the public and health professionals.

The STFM group on immunization education: shots online

Developed with support from the CDC, Shots (www.immunizationed.org/ShotsOnline.aspx) is a free point-of-care IIS that can be accessed online and is compatible with iPhone, iTouch, Android, Blackberry Storm, Palm Pre, or personal computer (PC). A downloadable version is available for Palm and Pocket PC handhelds. Shots contains

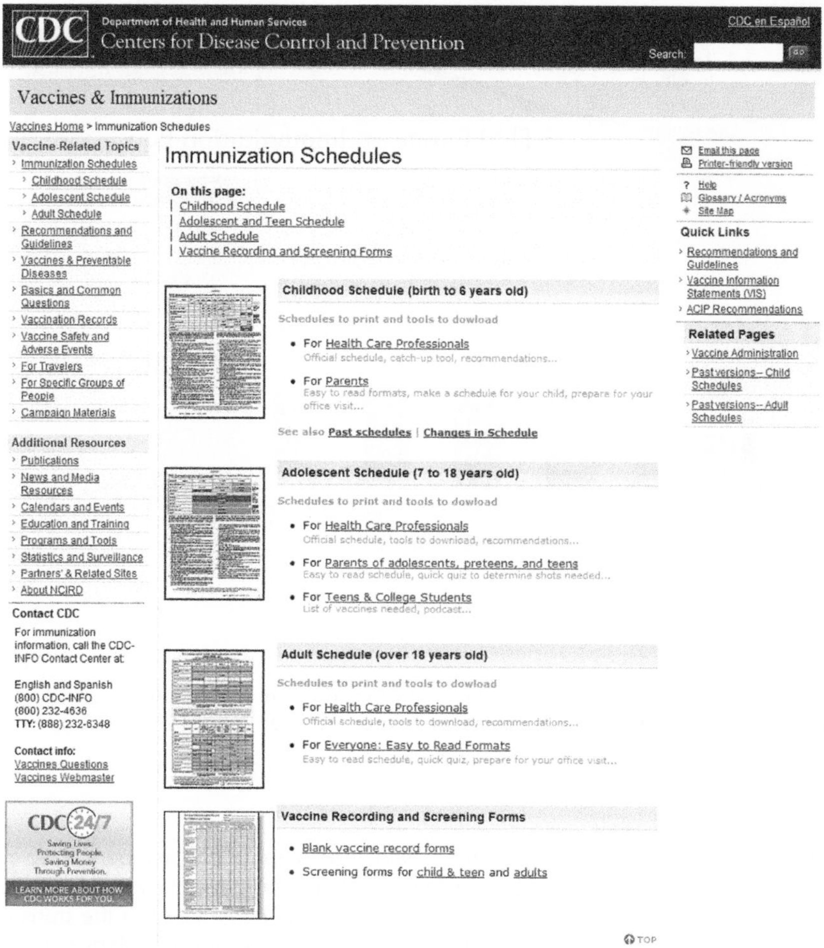

Fig. 3. CDC Immunization Schedules. (*Data from* Available at: http://www.cdc.gov/vaccines/recs/schedules/default.htm. Accessed August 28, 2011.)

the complete immunization schedules for children, teenagers, adults, and persons with special medical conditions (**Fig. 4**).

Information can be quickly viewed for each individual vaccine regarding immunization basics, high-risk indications, adverse reactions, contraindications, administration, catch-up schedules, and disease epidemiology and pictures. The Shots program is updated regularly, and users can request e-mail notification of new releases and updates.

AAP

Devoted to immunization information, this site (http://www.aap.org/immunization/about/about.html) is nicely designed and includes a family section and a pediatric provider section.

AAFP

The "Clinical and Research" section has an "Immunization" section with links to a variety of Web resources (http://www.aafp.org/online/en/home/clinical/immunizationres.html). The home page links to vaccine resources and reviews shortages and delays.

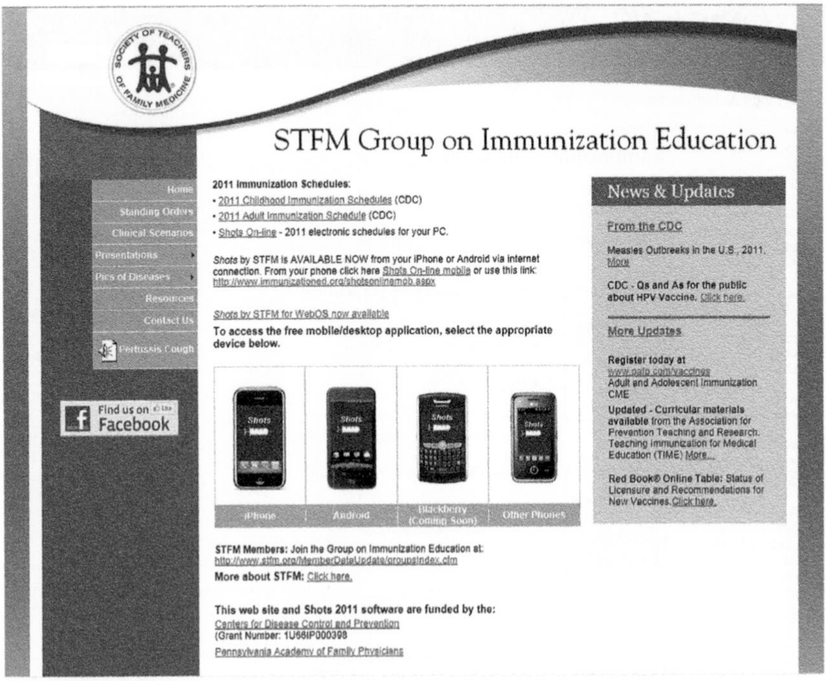

Fig. 4. Society of Teachers of Family Medicine Group on Immunization Education. (*Data from* Available at: http://www.immunizationed.org/. Accessed August 28, 2011.)

Manufacturers' web sites

A complete list of vaccine manufacturers, with addresses, phone numbers, Web site, and e-mail information, is available at the IAC Web site, http://www.immunize.org/resources/manufact_vax.asp. The manufacturers' Web sites assist in the transition from the ACIP schedules to the actual products used for vaccination. Many combination vaccines help to limit the number of injections; so, staying current with available products is paramount. Product circulars are updated almost immediately after any changes and remain a good source of information for any basic detail.

National Network for Immunization Information (NNii)

The National Network for Immunization Information (NNii, http://www.immunizationinfo.org/NNii) provides up-to-date information to health care professionals, the media, and the public, especially for parents, and quick access to state vaccine requirements. Each VPD quickly links to understanding the disease, available vaccines, history of the vaccine, who should and should not receive the vaccine, dose schedule, effectiveness of the vaccine, known side effects, related issues, key references, sources of additional information, and CDC information. NNii is an affiliation of the Infectious Diseases Society of America (IDSA), the Pediatric Infectious Diseases Society, the AAP, the American Nurses Association (ANA), the AAFP, the National Association of Pediatric Nurse Practitioners, the American College of Obstetricians and Gynecologists, the University of Texas Medical Branch, the Society for Adolescent Medicine, and the American Medical Association.

National Foundation for Infectious Diseases

The nonprofit National Foundation for Infectious Diseases (NFID) Web site (http://www.nfid.org/) presents fact sheets about a number of infectious diseases and vaccines and links to NFID-sponsored sites about adult immunization, the Childhood Influenza Immunization Coalition, an adolescent vaccination site, a STOP Meningitis site, and several resource centers on Medscape.

Medscape

Medscape (http://www.medscape.com/resource/vaccines) from WebMD provides health professionals medical information and educational tools. The Medscape Immunization Resource Center has an extensive collection of articles on child and adult immunizations, with information on specific diseases and links to useful sites. Registration for site access is free.

The National Vaccine Program Office and the National Vaccine Advisory Committee

The National Vaccine Program Office (http://www.hhs.gov/nvpo/index.html) is responsible for coordinating and ensuring collaboration among the many federal agencies involved in vaccine and immunization activities. The National Vaccine Advisory Committee (NVAC; http://www.hhs.gov/nvpo/nvac/index.html) advises the Director of the National Vaccine Program on program responsibilities. The NVAC Web site includes the committee's published reports on vaccine issues and safety.

Children's Hospital of Philadelphia

The Children's Hospital of Philadelphia's Vaccine Education Center provides accurate, comprehensive, and up-to-date information about vaccines and VPDs for parents and health care professionals (www.chop.edu). The center, through its videos, information tear sheets, and speaker programs, seeks to dispel common misconceptions and misinformation surrounding vaccines. The Center Director, Paul A. Offit, MD, is Chief of Infectious Diseases at The Children's Hospital of Philadelphia and is a leader in the effort to combat misinformation about vaccines.

The Institute for Vaccine Safety at the Johns Hopkins University School of Public Health

The Institute for Vaccine Safety provides an independent assessment of vaccines and vaccine safety to help guide decision makers and educate physicians, the public, and the media about key issues in vaccine safety, including information on the safety of vaccine additives, vaccine injury law, and recent news (http://www.vaccinesafety.edu/). The institute's goal is to work toward preventing disease using the safest vaccines possible. Legislative issues and personal and religious exemptions are also covered.

Google

The astonishingly accurate Flu Trends Web site (google.org/flutrends/) tracks influenza activity around the world based on the close relationship between how many people search for flu-related topics and how many people actually have flu symptoms. Searching on Google (http://www.google.com) can produce mixed results. Although the words immunization or immunizations produce consistently high-quality information, the terms vaccine or vaccination also bring up a large number of antivaccination sites in the top search results.[10,11] Google ranks sites by the number of other sites linked to it on the Internet. Antivaccination sites almost exclusively use the terms "vaccine" or "vaccination" and avoid the term "immunization" because investigators on these sites do not believe vaccines produce immunity. Although health care providers can distinguish between the two, patients may be confused by misinformation they find during such vaccine-related health searches.

Vaccine Adverse Event Reporting System

The Vaccine Adverse Event Reporting System site (http://vaers.hhs.gov/index) details reported reactions after immunization, some of which are actually linked to vaccines and some which are not. This site is open to the public, and anyone can report a vaccine reaction. The data are further analyzed to detect scientifically based important reactions. For example, some individuals reported that syncope followed vaccination with human papillomavirus vaccine. An analysis showed that 76% of episodes of syncope occurred in adolescents and that 80% of the reported syncope episodes occurred within 15 minutes of vaccine administration.[12] This analysis led to the recommendation that adults and adolescents be seated or lie down during vaccination and that after vaccination with human papillomavirus, diphtheria and reduced tetanus toxoids and acellular pertussis, or meningococcal vaccine, adolescents should be observed for 15 minutes to decrease the risk of injury from fainting.

FDA

The FDA site (http://www.fda.com/) presents a wealth of information about available immunizations, a key topic, and serves as a good source of vaccination information for interested patients. A search engine is available that leads to published articles about vaccine safety and various FDA newsletters. It is useful for confirming the accuracy of rumors about current vaccines.

Institute of medicine

Besides routine data, the Institute of Medicine Web site (http://www.iom.edu/) reports on racial and ethnic disparities in vaccine rates and provides information on travel vaccines.

Drug programs

Most drug programs cover available vaccines. Epocrates for handheld devices and phones gives information about individual vaccine products. An excellent source is the John Hopkins Antibiotic Guide at http://www.hopkinsguides.com/hopkins/, which has information about vaccines and VPDs.

NEWSLETTERS

Newsletters are convenient sources of up-to-date immunization information. Most can be delivered directly to the e-mail box.

Morbidity and Mortality Weekly Report (MMWR), from the CDC, is the quintessential comprehensive CDC publication. This publication often features information on immunization recommendations and on VPDs. *MMWR* can be viewed online at http://www.cdc.gov/mmwr/ or via updates sent directly to the readers' computer after submitting their e-mail address in the home page right column box entitled "Get Email Updates." Perusal of the 2011 general recommendations on immunization[13] takes the practitioner seeking excellence in vaccination to an extraordinary command of the topic.

The ANA puts out an electronic newsletter twice a month and features articles selected with nurses in mind, often stressing school health. The *ANA ImmuNews*is can be signed up at http://www.anaimmunize.org/.

The CDC newsletter, *Immunization Works*, at http://www.cdc.gov/vaccines/news/newsltrs/imwrks/, is published monthly. The information provided is nonproprietary and meant to be widely shared.

The IAC publishes weekly e-mail immunization information for health professionals, *IAC Express*, at http://www.immunize.org/express/. Subscription to this premier newsletter brings periodic e-mail messages about new and important immunization information. The newsletter, *Needle Tips*, which contains "Ask the Experts" with questions generated from practitioners, is downloadable from http://www.immunize.org or can be automatically sent to the reader as it is published.

The NNii Web site, http://www.immunizationinfo.org, provides the latest immunization news from both home and abroad. To subscribe to the newsletter scroll down to "News" on the right-hand side and click on "Subscribe."

The AAP publishes the *AAP Immunization Initiatives Newsletter* available at: http://www.aap.org/immunization/pediatricians/newsletters/.

CONFERENCES

National Meetings

National conferences offer a forum to interact directly with physicians, nurses, public health professionals, government and military personnel, and other stakeholders with interest in vaccination. The National Immunization Conference, the NFID Annual Conference on Vaccine Research, and the NFID Seasonal and Pandemic Influenza Conference are devoted to information on vaccines. Many continuing medical education (CME) conferences are likely to offer immunization education. One can also sign up to attend the ACIP meetings through the Web site.

National Immunization Conference

The CDC holds the National Immunization Conference every other year, last in 2011. The goals are to provide information that helps participants provide comprehensive immunization coverage for all age groups and explore innovative strategies for developing programs, policy, and research to promote immunization coverage for all age groups. The topics presented during 3 and a half days of plenary sessions and workshops include childhood immunization, adolescent immunization, adult immunization, assessment, barriers to vaccination, community and partnerships, cultural diversity, global immunization surveillance, health communications, health education, policy and legislation, new vaccines and vaccine development, VPDs, vaccine safety, and immunization registries. Registration is at http://www.cdc.gov/vaccines/events/nic/.

NFID

The NFID's Annual Conference on Vaccine Research at http://www.nfid.org/ has become the largest scientific meeting devoted exclusively to research on vaccines and associated technologies for disease prevention through immunization. The target audience for this conference is researchers and scientists, epidemiologists, microbiologists, immunologists, molecular biologists, nurses and nurse practitioners, pharmacologists, physicians in training, physicians, veterinarians, postgraduate fellows, public health officials, and vaccine, diagnostic, and device manufacturers. The NFID also sponsors CME courses on vaccinology and immunization-related subjects.

IDSA

The Seasonal and Pandemic Influenza Conference is a hybrid event with both in-person and virtual participants. The IDSA annual conference includes immunization-related presentations, but they are generally a small component of the conference that focuses on all aspects of a wide variety of infectious diseases. Sign up is at http://www.idsociety.org/.

The following conferences are likely to include presentations on immunizations but are not dedicated to immunization topics.

AAFP

The AAFP Annual Scientific Assembly attracts 4200 family physicians from around the country to this comprehensive educational event. Sign up is at http://www.aafp.org. The AAFP also sponsors a periodic conference on infant, child, and adolescent medicine that details immunization advances.

AAP

The AAP National Conference and Exhibit brings together health care professionals who care for infants, children, and adolescents. The conference offers CME, lifelong learning, and networking on a wide variety of pediatric medicine topics, including immunizations at http://www.aapexperience.org/.

ACP

The ACP's annual conference, Internal Medicine, is a comprehensive educational event in internal medicine, offering 260 courses. Immunization topics are included in the program at http://www.acponline.org/.

STFM

The Annual Spring Conference offers presentations focusing on best practices, new teaching technologies, emerging research, and public policy issues. This meeting is the most powerful networking forum for family medicine educators, with an attendance of more than 1000. Immunization topics may be included in the STFM's conferences at www.stfm.org.

OTHER SOURCES

Many local conferences at hospitals, medical societies, and universities or in the office are devoted to immunization practices and may offer the opportunity for easy interaction with the presenters. State articles of various specialties often offer live or recorded webinars on vaccine use through their home pages.

GROUPS FOR IMMUNIZATION CAMARADERIE

Local and national immunization coalitions offer networking possibilities for those interested in promoting immunizations. The Group on Immunization Education (GIE) of the STFM is dedicated to educating practicing physicians, residents, students, and affiliated health care personnel about VPDs and the importance of immunizations in prevention. The GIE facilitates the development of educational resources to disseminate new recommendations and information about vaccines to educators and practitioners.

The GIE produces Shots by STFM, a free immunization application for mobile phones and PCs to access immunization schedules and other critical information on immunizations at the point of care at http://www.Immunizationed.org or http://www.cdc.gov (see **Fig. 3**).

Local immunization coalitions are valuable resources to promote immunizations in their community. To locate a coalition in any particular area, the reader is suggested to search the Directory of Immunization Coalitions at: http://izcoalitions.org/, a project of the IAC. For example, immunization coalitions in Pennsylvania include the Allegheny County Immunization Coalition at http://www.ImmunizeAllegheny.org, which has a membership representing 50 organizations, including hospitals, universities, private practice physicians, school nurses, pharmacists, insurance carriers, vaccine manufacturers, and educators. This coalition is affiliated with and funded by the Allegheny County Health Department. The coalition provides educational and networking opportunities for its members and reaches out to the community to provide immunization resources. The goal of the coalition is community immunity. The Pennsylvania Immunization Coalition at http://www.immunizepa.org/ is an organization of volunteers with interest in advancing timely and effective immunization for all Pennsylvania residents. The leaders of the coalition act as liaisons, sharing information with many local immunization coalitions in Pennsylvania.

EXPERT OPINION

Expert advice can be obtained from many local experts and state health department personnel who can be contacted for specific questions. The CDC may be contacted at (800) 232-4636 and has an online site to which questions can be submitted at http://www.cdc.gov/vaccines/about/contact/nipinfo_contact_form.htm. CDC's travel information phone line is 1-877-394-8747. Frequently answered questions are available at CDC's Web site, and the IAC has a useful "Q&A" column on their Web site http://www.immunize.org/askexperts/ and in "Needle Tips."

VACCINE TEXTBOOKS AND JOURNALS

Textbooks provide authoritative sources of information on immunization but must be updated online to stay current. The standard full-detail text, *Vaccines*,[14] with1725 pages and 76 articles, covers nearly every aspect of vaccine science and policy. Many consider it to be the bible of vaccine science.

Perhaps the most well-known text for clinical use is the 984-page "Redbook: 2009 Report on the Committee on Infectious Diseases" of the AAP.[15] This text addresses the spectrum of infectious diseases that affect children and has an online version at http://aapredbook.aappublications.org/.

A useful and low-cost text is the "Epidemiology and Prevention of Vaccine-Preventable Diseases," also known as the "Pink Book."[16] Articles that address the common vaccines and administration can be downloaded for free at http://www.cdc.gov/vaccines/pubs/pinkbook/. It is a practical and useful guide with extensive appendices.

For travel vaccines, CDC's "Health Information for International Travel,"[17] also called the "Yellow Book" is available free at http://wwwnc.cdc.gov/travel/yellowbook/2010/table-of-contents.aspx.

The "Vaccine Handbook, A Practical Guide for Clinicians" by Marshall,[18] is another useful resource about vaccines across the life span.

Some texts are helpful for parents or patients with questions about vaccines. Two such texts are "Vaccines: What Every Parent Should Know"[19] and "Vaccinating your Child: Questions and Answers for the Concerned Parent."[20]

The journal *Vaccine* is devoted to its title topic. Periodic reviews are available in the *American Family Physician*, *New England Journal of Medicine*, *American Journal of Preventive Medicine*, *Pediatrics, the Annuals of Internal Medicine*, and other publications. Use of a search journal engine can locate the many articles on a specific topic.

OUR FAVORITES

For answering clinical questions rapidly at the point of care, our favorites are Shots (www.immunizationed.org) and the CDC schedules. Current detailed information can be found at the CDC's Web site (www.cdc.gov/vaccines) and the "Pink Book," and, for influenza, the CDC's flu Web site (www.cdc.gov/flu). Sample forms, VISs in a variety of languages, and pictures of VPD can be found at the IAC's Web site www.immunize.org. We feel interested persons should sign up for *MMWR*, e-mails from the CDC, and *IAC Express*. For conferences, we advise the National Immunization Conference or attending a local immunization coalition meeting that we have found to be outstanding.

SUMMARY

Next to clean water and sewage control, immunizations are at the top of all the scientific advances in the arena of public health over the past decade and century.[2] The power of vaccination to save lives and reduce morbidity is unmatched. Every primary care provider should latch onto this valuable tool to promote health and well-being and continue self-education to better serve their charges. This article reviews some of the most trustworthy sources to achieve that end.

REFERENCES

1. Maciosek MV, Coffield AB, Edwards NM, et al. Priorities among effective clinical preventive services. Am J Prev Med 2006;31:52–61.
2. Centers for Disease Control and Prevention. Ten great public health achievements—United States 2001–2010. MMWR Morb Mortal Wkly Rep 2011;60(19): 619–23.
3. Kinrix product circular. Available at: http://us.gsk.com/products/assets/us_kinrix.pdf. Accessed August 28, 2011.
4. Offit P. Deadly choices. New York City (NY): Basic Books; 2011.
5. Centers for Disease Control and Prevention. IIS/What is IIS? Available at: http://www.cdc.gov/vaccines/programs/iis/what-iis.htm. Accessed March 3, 2011.
6. Centers for Disease Control and Prevention (CDC). Progress in immunization information systems—United States, 2009. MMWR Morb Mortal Wkly Rep 2011; 60(1):10–2.
7. Centers for Disease Control and Prevention. Progress in immunization information system—United States, 2008. MMWR Morb Mortal Wkly Rep 2010;59(5):133–5.
8. Hinman AR, Ross DA. Immunization registries can be building blocks for national health information systems. Health Aff (Millwood) 2010;29(4):676–82.
9. Centers for Medicare & Medicaid Services. Electronic health records incentive programs. Available at: https://www.cms.gov/ehrincentiveprograms/. Accessed March 3, 2011.
10. Wolfe RM, Sharp LK. Vaccination or immunization? The impact of search terms on the Internet. J Health Commun 2005;10(6):537–51.
11. Zimmerman RK, Wolfe RM, Fox DE, et al. Vaccine criticism on the World Wide Web. J Med Internet Res 2005;7(2):e17.
12. Kata A. A postmodern Pandora's box: anti-vaccination misinformation on the Internet. Vaccine 2010;28(7):1709–16.
13. Kroger AT, Sumaya CV, Pickering LK, et al. General recommendations on immunization: recommendations of the Advisory Committee on Immunization Practices (ACIP): recommendations and reports. MMWR Morb Mortal Wkly Rep 2011; 60(RRo2):1–60. Available at: http://www.cdc.gov/mmwr/preview/mmwrhtml/rr6002a1.htm?s_cid=rr6002a1_w. Accessed August 28, 2011.
14. Plotkin SA, Orenstein W, Offit PA. Vaccines. 5th edition. Cambridge (MA): Saunders Elsevier; 2008.

15. Pickering LK, Baker CJ, Kimberlin DW, et al. 2009 red book: report of the Committee on Infectious Diseases. 28th edition. Elk Grove Village (IL): AAP; 2009.
16. Atkinson W, Wolfe C, Hamborsky J, et al. Epidemiology and prevention of vaccine-preventable diseases. 12th edition. Atlanta (GA): National Center for Immunization and Respiratory Diseases, Centers for Disease Control and Prevention; 2011.
17. Brunette GW, Kozarsky PE, Magill AJ. CDC health information for international travel 2010: the yellow book. Cambridge (MA): Elsevier; 2009. (New edition due summer of 2012).
18. Marshall GS. The vaccine handbook: a practical guide for clinicians. 3rd edition. West Islip (NY): Professional Communications, Inc; 2010.
19. Offit PA, Bell LM. Vaccines: what every parent should know. 2nd edition. Hoboken (NJ): Wiley; 1999.
20. Humiston SG, Good CE. Vaccinating your child: questions and answers for the concerned parent. Atlanta (GA): Peachtree Publishers; 2000.

Q & A: Patient to Physician FAQs: Answers to Common Patient Questions About Vaccinations

Kathryn P. Trayes, MD[a,*], Kathryn M. Conniff, MD[b]

KEYWORDS

• Questions • Answers • Vaccinations

Q: WHAT ARE SOME OF THE ADVERSE EVENTS ASSOCIATED WITH VACCINATIONS AND WHAT ARE THE ABSOLUTE CONTRAINDICATIONS FOR VACCINE ADMINISTRATION?

A: Large-scale vaccination programs have changed the face of health care in the last few decades. In 1980, the World Health Organization declared that smallpox had been eradicated and polio eradication was an achievable goal. Immunizations have reduced the incidence of many diseases, including measles, mumps, rubella, tetanus, and polio, in the United Stated by more than 95% compared with the prevaccine era.[1] However, now that these diseases are less prevalent, attention has shifted from the consequences of the disease to vaccine-associated adverse events. Because vaccines are often mandated and administered to healthy people, and in part because of the way vaccinations are portrayed in the media, there is a widespread public lack of understanding and trust in vaccinations.[2] As clinicians navigate the continuously evolving complexities of vaccine administration, managing individual patient risk factors and educating the public about adverse reactions are critical to obtaining public confidence in vaccine safety.

Adverse events from vaccines range from minor to life threatening. Minor, expected reactions include irritation at the site of injection (swelling, redness, and soreness), low-grade fever, and malaise. These reactions usually last for a few days or less

[a] Department of Family and Community Medicine, Thomas Jefferson University Hospital, Jefferson Medical College of Thomas Jefferson University, 1020 Locust Street, Suite 157, Philadelphia, PA 19107, USA
[b] Department of Family Medicine, University of Maryland School of Medicine, 29 South Paca Street, Baltimore, MA 21201, USA
* Corresponding author.
E-mail address: Kathryn.Trayes@jefferson.edu

Prim Care Clin Office Pract 38 (2011) 763–776
doi:10.1016/j.pop.2011.07.012
0095-4543/11/$ – see front matter Published by Elsevier Inc.

and resolve without sequelae.[3] A later finding associated with vaccine administration that often prompts patients to visit a physician is a delayed-type hypersensitivity reaction that results in an injection site nodule. These patients should be counseled that most of these nodules resolve over time, although it can take several months, and that nodules are not a contraindication for future vaccination.[4]

More serious reactions include severe hypersensitivity reactions and anaphylaxis. These reactions may be caused by the vaccine antigen itself or components used in the manufacturing of the vaccine (eg, residual animal protein, gelatin, preservatives, or stabilizers). Egg protein is used in the preparation of influenza and yellow fever vaccines; however, most patients with egg allergies are able to tolerate these vaccines without difficulty. Although measles, mumps, and rabies vaccines are grown in chick embryos, they contain no egg protein and can be administered to patients with egg allergies.[5]

Gelatin is used by some manufacturers in the production of the Japanese encephalitis, varicella, and measles, mumps, rubella (MMR) vaccines. It is often identified as the culprit in hypersensitivity reactions to the MMR vaccine.[6] Thimerosal, a preservative that contains mercury, has been a source of great controversy. Even although the amount of mercury is minimal, most manufacturers have removed thimerosal from the vaccine production process.[7] Aluminum and phenoxyethanol are 2 other preservatives used in vaccines that can cause hypersensitivity reactions. Residual yeast proteins may be found in the hepatitis B and human papillomavirus (HPV) vaccines.[1]

Contrary to popular belief, most patients with suspected allergies or even anaphylaxis to vaccines or their components may receive vaccines safely. Patients who report an allergy to vaccine components should be referred to an allergist for immediate-skin type testing to determine if vaccine administration is appropriate.[8] For patients who have experienced anaphylactic reactions to vaccines or their components, evaluation with skin testing is warranted in an attempt to determine the culprit allergen.[9] Despite positive skin testing, the vaccine may still be administered in graded doses with 15-minute intervals under direct medical supervision.[10]

In patients who experience an adverse reaction to a vaccine with recommended subsequent doses, IgG antibody levels should be measured to determine the presence or absence of seroprotection. If the levels are appropriate, additional doses may be withheld despite the fact that the magnitude and duration of immunity may be decreased.[11]

Besides anaphylactic reactions, specific serious adverse reactions associated with certain vaccines may be absolute contraindications for the administration of future doses. For example, encephalopathy has been associated with MMR and pertussis vaccines.

Live vaccines may cause vaccine-induced illness and special attention needs to be given to each patient's immune and pregnancy status. The live vaccines include bacillus Calmette-Guérin (BCG), intranasal influenza, oral polio, MMR, rotavirus, oral typhoid smallpox, varicella, and yellow fever. These vaccines are contraindicated in patients with immunosuppression, either from humoral or cellular immune deficiency or immunosuppression caused by medications such as steroids.[1] The duration and dose of steroid treatment considered to be a contraindication to vaccination with live viruses is controversial, and the risks and benefits of such vaccinations should be reviewed on an individual case basis.[1] The only live vaccine that cannot be administered to close contacts of immunocompromised individuals is oral polio.[12]

Live vaccinations are contraindicated in pregnancy and women should be counseled to avoid becoming pregnant for at least 1 month after receiving a live vaccine because of the theoretic risk of transmitting the live agent to the fetus (see **Table 1** for a general overview of the Advisory Committee on Immunization Practices [ACIP] guidelines for vaccination of pregnant women).[13] If a live-virus vaccine is inadvertently

Table 1
Guidelines for vaccination of pregnant women

	Vaccine	Should be Considered if Otherwise Indicated	Contraindicated
Routine	Hepatitis A		
	Hepatitis B	X	
	HPV		
	Influenza (inactivated)	Recommended	
	Influenza (live attenuated influenza virus)[a]		X
	Measles[a]		X
	Meningococcal (meningococcal conjugate vaccine 4 [MPSV4])		
	Mumps[a]		X
	Pneumococcal		
	Polio (inactivated poliovirus vaccine)		
	Rubella[a]		X
	Tetanus-diphtheria	X	
	Tetanus-diphtheria-pertussis		
	Varicella[a]		X
Travel and other	Anthrax		
	BCG[a]		X
	Japanese encephalitis		
	Meningococcal (MPSV4)	X	
	Rabies	X	
	Typhoid		
	Vaccinia[a]		X
	Yellow fever[a]		
	Zoster[a]		X

[a] Live attenuated vaccines.

Adapted from Center for Disease Control and Prevention. Guidelines for vaccinating pregnant women from recommendations of the Advisory Committee on Immunization Practices (ACIP). Atlanta (GA): Centers for Disease Control and Prevention; 2007.

given to a pregnant woman, she should be counseled about the potential effects on the fetus, but it is not an indication for termination. With the exception of smallpox, no vaccines are contraindicated in breastfeeding mothers.[14]

To maintain public confidence in immunizations for the continued prevention of vaccine-preventable diseases, health care providers must keep updated on vaccine dosing schedules, changing contraindications for vaccine administration, and recommendations for storing and administering vaccines correctly. Health care providers should educate patients on benefits and risks of immunizations and ensure patients are aware of expected, minor reactions to vaccinations and which reactions require follow-up care.

Q: WHAT ARE THE RISKS AND BENEFITS OF GIVING MMR AND VARICELLA VACCINES SEPARATELY VERSUS COMBINED IN THE MEASLES, MUMPS, RUBELLA, AND VARICELLA VACCINE? DOES THE MEASLES, MUMPS, RUBELLA, AND VARICELLA VACCINE CONFER AN INCREASED RISK FOR FEBRILE SEIZURES?

A: The ACIP recommends a 2-dose vaccine schedule to prevent measles, mumps, rubella, and varicella (MMRV), with the first dose administration at age 12 to 15 months and the second dose at age 4 to 6 years.[15,16] MMRV was first licensed by the Food and Drug Administration in 2005. Initially, the ACIP of the Centers for Disease Control (CDC) recommended using the combination vaccine over MMR and varicella separately for both the first and second doses. However, in February 2008, preliminary data from 2 postlicensure studies suggested a 2.3-fold increased risk of febrile seizures in children aged 12 to 23 months who received the first dose of the MMRV vaccine compared with children of the same age who received the first doses of MMR and varicella as separate injections at the same visit.[17–19] The increased risk did not apply to children aged 4 to 6 years after receiving the second dose. This finding was believed to be related to the window of vulnerability for febrile seizures; 97% occur in children less than 4 years of age.[20]

Between 2% and 5% of children between birth and 60 months experience at least 1 febrile seizure.[21] The peak incidence is between 14 and 18 months. Febrile seizures have a good prognosis and most children recover completely. Approximately one-third of children who have a febrile seizure experience another in the future.[22] Children who experience a febrile seizure after administration of the MMR or MMRV vaccine are not more likely than children who have febrile seizures unrelated to vaccine administration to develop epilepsy or neurodevelopmental disorders.[23–25] However, 1 study suggests children who experience a vaccine-related febrile seizure are at increased risk of experiencing additional isolated febrile seizures.[24]

Based on these results, the ACIP changed its recommendation in June 2009 to include a personal or family history of febrile seizures as a precaution for use of the combination MMRV vaccine. The CDC now recommends the separate administration of the MMR and varicella vaccines for the first dose in children age 12 to 47 months. For the second dose (age 15 months–12 years) or the first dose in children 48 months or older, the MMRV vaccine is preferable, but it is acceptable to give MMR and varicella vaccines separately.[18]

Q: WHAT IS VARICELLA BREAKTHROUGH DISEASE, AND WHAT IS ITS SIGNIFICANCE?

A: Varicella breakthrough disease is a case of wild-type varicella occurring in a person more than 42 days after vaccination.[26] From 70% to 75% of these cases are milder than wild-type varicella (without fever, less than 50 lesions, maculopapular instead of vesicular, and shorter in duration) in an unimmunized individual.[27] Before the introduction of routine vaccination against varicella, 100 to 150 people died of the infection yearly, but only 2 deaths have been reported from breakthrough disease; both were children undergoing treatment with steroids at the time of infection.[26] The breakthrough rate is 3 times lower in patients who have received 2 doses of the vaccine compared with those who have received only 1 dose.[28] Breakthrough disease with less than 50 lesions is one-third as contagious as varicella in unvaccinated individuals, but may be equally transmissible in cases where there are more than 50 lesions.[29]

As the incidence of varicella continues to decrease and the proportion of milder cases increases, the disease has become increasingly difficult to recognize clinically. In 1 study, only 75% of unvaccinated children aged 1 to 4 years with a reported positive history of varicella disease were immune by serologic testing, compared with 89% of children between the ages of 5 to 14 years, 99% between ages 15 and 19 years, and 100% between ages 20 and 29 years.[30] Thus, self-reported history of varicella disease or breakthrough disease is not sufficient evidence for immunity in people born after 1980; the ACIP requires that a health care provider diagnose the disease or verify disease history in this age-group by either documenting an epidemiologic link to a laboratory-confirmed or typical case of varicella or by obtaining serology. The same requirement holds true for health care workers, pregnant women, and immunocompromised individuals. If documentation cannot be obtained or serologic testing indicates lack of immunity, a 2-dose vaccination series is indicated.[26]

Q: IS THE HPV VACCINE INDICATED IN WOMEN WHO HAVE ALREADY BEEN INFECTED WITH HPV?

A: Genital HPV is the most common sexually transmitted infection in the United States. There are more than 30 HPV strains that cause benign, low-grade cervical changes to squamous cell or adenocarcinoma. Seventy percent of cervical cancers worldwide are caused by HPV strains 16 and 18. These 2 strains account for 68% of squamous cell cervical cancer and 83% of adenocarcinoma, 76% of vulvar intraepithelial neoplasia, and 42% of vulvar carcinoma. Ninety percent of anogenital warts are caused by HPV 6 and 11.[31]

It is estimated that 40% of women acquire at least 1 strain of HPV within 16 months of sexarche.[32] Greater than 80% of sexually active women have acquired HPV by the age of 50 years.[33] The incidence of HPV rises with increasing number of partners. HPV is found in 14% of women age 18 to 25 years with 1 lifetime sexual partner, and greater than 31.5% of women with more than 3 sexual partners.[34] Most HPV infections are asymptomatic and transient, 70% of new HPV infections clear within 1 year, and 90% of new HPV infections clear within 2 years. Because most HPV infections are transient, HPV DNA is often detected for only a short period.[35]

Further complicating the detection of HPV is the inability to clinically differentiate between viral strains.[36] Polymerase chain reaction (PCR) assays are used in epidemiologic studies along with HPV serologic assays to distinguish between HPV types.[37] The only test approved in the United States to detect HPV in the clinical setting is the hybrid capture 2 high-risk HPV DNA test. This test uses liquid nucleic acid hybridization to detect 13 high-risk types of HPV and reports samples as positive or negative and is therefore not type-specific.[38]

In June 2006, Merck developed Gardasil, a quadrivalent vaccine, which provides protection against HPV types 6, 11, 16, and 18. This vaccine is licensed for women ages 9 to 26 years, with the target age being 11 to 12 years.[38] In October 2009, Cervarix, a bivalent vaccine that protects against HPV 16 and 18, was released by GlaxoSmithKline and approved for women aged 10 to 26 years.[39] The recommended vaccination schedule is that administered at 0, 2, and 6 months; however, this schedule can be extended if the patients are unable to be seen in the office (ie, patients who are away at college). Overall, both vaccines have been shown to have good safety records, excellent immunogenicity, and high efficacy against cervical precancers.[35]

Data from the ongoing Females United to Unilaterally Reduce Endo/Ectocervical Disease (FUTURE) trial shows the vaccine is highly effective in reducing the occurrence of high-grade cervical intraepithelial neoplasia and a significant reduction in the incidence of HPV-associated anogenital disease in women who have no evidence of infection with the types of HPV included in the vaccine.[40,41] In the 25% of women enrolled in these trials who had serologic or PCR evidence of previous or current infection with HPV-6, HPV-11, HPV-16, or HPV-18, there was no evidence that vaccination altered the course of disease or infection present before the administration of the first dose.

A 2007 study examined the efficacy of Gardasil in women with virological evidence of HPV infection before vaccine administration. The population group studied was a cohort of women from the FUTURE trial who were infected with 1 to 3 HPV vaccine types at enrollment. The study concluded that this population of women benefited from the administration of Gardasil because it provided protection from infections caused by the HPV types to which they were naive. The findings of this study led to the FUTURE II Study Group recommendation that prescreening for the presence of HPV infection before giving the vaccination is unnecessary because infection with all 4 HPV vaccine types is rare. In addition, women who are infected with 1 to 3 of the HPV types targeted by the vaccine may be at high risk for acquisition of infection with the remaining HPV types.[42] Thus, universal catch-up immunization with the HPV vaccine is reasonable, regardless of current HPV status.

Q: IS IT SAFE TO ADMINISTER THE HERPES ZOSTER VACCINATION TO A PATIENT WHO HAS ALREADY HAD SHINGLES?

A: Herpes zoster, or shingles, results from the reactivation of latent varicella zoster virus.[43] This reactivation can occur decades after the initial infection. It most commonly occurs in older adults, with a peak incidence in individuals older than 75 years. Approximately 1 in 3 persons develop zoster during their lifetime.[44] Herpes zoster often starts as erythematous papules that evolve into pustular vesicles that can then become hemorrhagic. In immunocompetent patients, these lesions generally start to crust by 3 to 5 days and completely crust over by 7 to 10 days, at which point they are no longer infectious.[45] This rash is preceded by pain in 75% of patients and it is often accompanied by neuropathic pain, allodynia, and severe pruritis.

Sequelae of herpes zoster include postherpetic neuralgia, uveitis, zoster keratitis, zoster ophthalmicus, motor neuropathy, and cellulitis. Postherpetic neuralgia is the most common complication of herpes zoster, and discomfort associated with this condition can be disabling, severely compromising the patient's quality of life.[46] Postherpetic neuralgia is defined by at least 90 days of documented pain; however, the pain may persist for years. The incidence of this condition increases with age. As many as 60% to 70% of people older than 60 years who have herpes zoster develop postherpetic neuralgia.[47]

The zoster vaccine, Zostavax, developed by Merck, was licensed in the United States in 2006.[48] Contraindications for the vaccine include pregnancy, leukemia, lymphomas or other malignancies affecting the bone marrow or lymphatic systems, primary and acquired immunodeficiency states such as human immunodeficiency virus (HIV) infection, and immunosuppressive therapy.[44]

The Shingles Prevention Study evaluated the efficacy of Zostavax in a double-blind, randomized, placebo-controlled trial involving 38,345 healthy adults 60 years and older. Participants had a history of varicella and no reported history of herpes zoster. The study concluded that Zostavax reduces the risk of developing zoster by 51.3%. It also showed that the vaccine was 66.5% effective in preventing postherpetic neuralgia.[49]

A randomized, double-blind, placebo-controlled crossover, multicenter study was conducted in the United States between May 2006 and July 2007 to examine the safety, tolerability, and immunogenicity of the zoster vaccine administered to patients with a history of herpes zoster. The results confirmed that the zoster vaccine is safe and immunogenic when administered to persons with a previous history of herpes zoster.[50] Thus, unless contraindicated, The ACIP recommends routine vaccination for all patients age 60 years or order, regardless of previous history of herpes zoster infection.[51]

Q: WHO SHOULD BE SCREENED FOR HEPATITIS B VIRUS? WHO SHOULD BE VACCINATED? WHAT IS A VACCINE NONRESPONDER?

A: Hepatitis B virus (HBV) is a DNA virus in the Hepadnaviridae family. It enters a susceptible person's liver through the bloodstream, and replicates primarily in the liver. The virus can be asymptomatic or symptomatic, and have an acute or chronic course.[52]

Acute hepatitis B usually has an insidious onset and is commonly mild. Infants and young children are often completely asymptomatic.[53] Those who are symptomatic may experience malaise, nausea, vomiting, anorexia, abdominal pain, and jaundice.[54] The overall mortality of acute HBV is 0.5% to 1.5%, with the highest occurrence in adults more than 60 years of age.[55]

Most of the burden of HBV is caused by the sequelae of chronic disease, which occurs in 90% of infected infants, 30% of children between ages 1 and 5 years, and less than 5% of infected persons older than 5 years. Chronically infected individuals serve as the major reservoir for HBV transmission.[56,57]

Interpretation of serologic markers can be challenging (**Table 2**). The presence of hepatitis B surface antigen (HbsAg) indicates an ongoing HBV infection. It is present an average of 30 days after exposure and wanes after the resolution of an acute infection typically within 3 to 4 months. HBsAg continues to be present in chronic infection.[58] Anti-hepatitis B core (anti-HBc) appears at symptom onset, usually in correlation with alanine transaminase (ALT) abnormalities. Anti-HBs usually indicates immunity from HBV and appears during resolution of acute infection or after vaccination. HB e antigen (HBeAg) correlates with high levels of viral replication and is therefore present in the serum of individuals who are highly infective.[59,60]

HBV transmission can occur through mucosal or percutaneous exposure to infected blood, serum, saliva, and semen.[61,62] HBV is stable at room temperature and can remain viable for at least 7 days on environmental surfaces.[63]

The 2 routes of HBV transmission in infants and children are vertical transmission from infected mothers (perinatally) and horizontal transmission from infected household contacts.[64] HBV is not transmitted through breast milk.[65] Risk factors for infection in adolescents and adults are high-risk sexual activity and injection drug use.[55]

Routine immunization of children against HBV began in 1991. During 1990 to 2004, the overall incidence of acute HBV decreased by 75%, from 8.5/100,000 to 2.1/100,000.[64] The vaccine has prevented an estimated 6800 perinatal infections and an additional 18,700 infections annually in children less than age 11 years.[66] Immigrants

Table 2
Interpretation of serologic tests for hepatitis B infection

HBsAg	Anti-HBc (Total)	Anti-HBc (IgM)	Anti-HBs	Interpretation
–	–	–	–	Never infection
+	–	–	–	Early acute infection; transient (up to 18 days) after vaccination
+	+	+	–	Acute infection
–	+	+	–	Resolving acute infection
+	+	–	–	Chronic infection
–	+	–	–	False-positive (ie, susceptible); past infection; low-level chronic infection; passive transfer to infant born to HBsAg-positive mother
–	–	–	+	Immune if concentration $\geq$10 mIU/mL; passive transfer after HBIG administration

Adapted from Mast EE, Margolis HS, Fiore AE. A comprehensive immunization strategy to eliminate transmission of hepatitis B virus infection in the United States. Recommendations of the Advisory Committee on Immunization Practices (ACIP) Part I: immunization of infants, children, and adolescents. MMWR Recomm Rep 2005;54(RR-16):1–31.

from endemic countries contribute disproportionately to the burden of chronic HBV in the United States.[64]

HBV prophylaxis is accomplished through the administration of either the HBV vaccine or hepatitis B immunoglobulin (HBIG). The active ingredient of the vaccine is HBsAg,[67] Primary vaccination in infants and children involves 3 intramuscular doses of the vaccine at birth, 1 to 2 months, and 6 to 18 months.[68] HBIG is used in combination with the HBV vaccine for postexposure prophylaxis (except in hepatitis vaccine nonresponders, in which case it is used alone; see later discussion). HBIG is harvested from donors whose blood contains high concentrations of anti-HBs (and the absence of HBsAg). It gives the recipient passively acquired anti-HBs, and thus temporary (3–6 months) protection from HBV infection.[64]

Successful vaccination is believed to confer at least 22 years of protection from HBV.[69] However, a small proportion (5%–15%) of those who receive the primary 3-dose series do not develop hepatitis B surface antibody (HbsAb).[70] Patients who fall in this category should first be tested to rule out infection (ie, HBsAg positivity), and should then receive a second 3-dose series. Between 30% and 50% of those who fail to respond to the first 3-dose series respond to a second series.[71,72] Those who fail to respond after the second 3-dose series are considered vaccine nonresponders, and are vulnerable to infection. They should be counseled regarding precautions to prevent infection and the need to receive HBIG immediately and again 1 month after known or probable exposure to HBV.

Seroprotection is less likely in individuals with diabetes and immunocompromised states and declines with aging.[72] The nonresponse rate is 33% in adults more than age 60 years and only 50% in adults with diabetes, compared with less than 10% in healthy individuals less than age 40 years.[73,74] The ACIP recommends testing for immunity after vaccination in these populations and those at high risk of exposure (eg, health care workers).

If a person reports risk factors, health care providers should screen for infection before vaccination by obtaining HBsAg. HbsAb, or hepatitis B core antibody should also be obtained in cases of unknown vaccination history and to ascertain susceptibility to infection (**Table 3**).[75]

To ensure vaccination against those at risk for HBV infection, health care providers should provide information to all adults about the benefits of HBV vaccination and recommend it for the following individuals: adults who report risk factors, susceptible household, sexual, and needle-sharing contacts of HBsAg-positive persons, and anyone receiving services at sexually transmitted disease (STD) clinics, HIV/AIDS counseling and testing centers, clinics targeting men who have sex with men, correctional facilities, and drug abuse treatment centers.[72]

Q: HOW SHOULD PATIENTS WHO ARE HESITANT TO RECEIVE THE INFLUENZA VACCINE BE COUNSELED?

A: There are 7 common reasons why patients refuse the influenza vaccine, most based on widespread misconceptions. The prospect of convincing patients with such deep-rooted beliefs to agree to the vaccine can seem daunting and even futile. By providing patients with evidence-based answers to their specific concerns, physicians may convince patients to receive the vaccine.

1. "But I'm healthy, and I've never gotten the flu in the past."

Patients often believe that healthy individuals are at low risk for contracting the virus. It is true that certain populations are at higher risk of complications (eg, pregnant

Table 3
Populations recommended or required for routine testing for chronic hepatitis infection

Population	Population-specific Testing Considerations
Persons born in region regions of high and intermediate HBV endemicity	Test for HBsAg, regardless of vaccination status in country of origin
US-born persons not vaccinated as infants whose parents were born in regions of high HBV endemicity	Test for HBsAg, regardless of maternal HBsAg status
Injection drug users	Test for HBsAg, anti-HBc, and anti-HBs to identify infection and susceptibility Administer first vaccine dose at same visit as testing Susceptible persons should complete a 3-dose vaccine series
Men who have sex with men	Test for HBsAg, anti-HBc, and anti-HBs to identify infection and susceptibility Administer first vaccine dose at same visit as testing Susceptible people should complete a 3-dose vaccine series
Persons requiring immunosuppressive or chemotherapy	Test for HBsAg, anti-HBc, and anti-HBs Because of the increased risk of fulminant hepatitis in chronically infected persons and risk for reactivation in persons with resolved infection, treat HBsAg-positive persons and monitor HBc-positive persons for signs of liver disease
Persons with increased aspartate aminotransferase/ALT of unknown cause	Test for HBsAg as part of a complete medical evaluation, including testing for other hepatitis viruses
Blood, plasma, organ, tissue, or semen donors	Test for HBsAg, anti-HBc, and HBV DNA to prevent transmission to recipients
Hemodialysis patients	Test for HBsAg, anti-HBc, and anti-HBs on admission Vaccinate all susceptible patients and revaccinate when serum anti-HBs decreases less than 10 mIU/mL Cohort HBsAg-positive patients Vaccine nonresponders should be screened for HBsAg monthly
Pregnant women	Test for HBsAg, preferably in first trimester If HBsAg result is not available or mother is at risk for infection during pregnancy, test for HBsAg at the time of admission for delivery
Infants born to HBsAg-positive mothers	Administer vaccine and HBIG within 12 hours of delivery Test for HBsAg and anti-HBs 1–2 months after completion of the 3-dose vaccine series to assess effectiveness of postexposure prophylaxis

Adapted from CDC. Recommendations for identification and public health management of persons with chronic hepatitis B virus infection. MMWR 2008;5(RR-8):1–20.

women, people with chronic medical conditions, young children, and elderly people) but even healthy people can become seriously ill from influenza. From 5% to 20% of healthy Americans contract the virus each year.[76]

2. "The flu isn't that big a deal."

There is a widespread lack of awareness that the influenza virus can cause serious illness, hospitalization, and even death. Influenza is characterized by the sudden onset of fever, chills, malaise, cough, rhinorrhea, congestion, myalgias, headache, fatigue, and less commonly, vomiting and diarrhea.[77] Recovery from even uncomplicated cases of the flu can take up to 2 weeks, and usually results in a significant number of missed work or school days. Complications of influenza include pneumonia, bronchitis, sinusitis, and otitis media, and the virus can exacerbate underlying asthma, chronic obstructive pulmonary disease, and congestive heart failure.

Flu severity varies from season to season. A study conducted by the CDC from 1979 to 2001 reported that an average of more than 200,000 people in the United States are hospitalized each year for flu-related complications.[77] Between 1976 and 2007, estimates of flu-related deaths ranged from 3000 to 49,000. Ninety percent of those deaths occurred in individuals aged 65 years and older.

3. "The flu vaccine makes me sick."

The influenza vaccine cannot cause the flu. The intramuscular vaccine is a killed virus, and the most common side effects are discomfort at the vaccination site and low-grade fever. The intranasal vaccine is an attenuated virus, and can cause rhinorrhea, cough, sore throat, or congestion. Patients should be reminded that these side effects are temporary and mild compared with the flu itself, which can result in multiple missed days of work, hospitalization, and even death.[76]

4. "I got the flu vaccine last year, but I still got the flu."

Patients often falsely attribute past experiences of falling ill after vaccination to the vaccine itself. Many nonflu viruses circulate during influenza season, so it is common for recently vaccinated individuals to become ill from viruses that cause similar symptoms. In addition, it is possible to contract the flu in the 2-week interval between the time of vaccination and when antibody protection is fully established. The vaccine protects only against the 3 strains predicted to cause the most illness each year, so vaccinated persons are still vulnerable if they are exposed to other strains not included in the vaccine.[76]

5. "It's too late."

A lack of understanding of appropriate timing of vaccination results in patients refusing the vaccine during the nonwinter months. Influenza season usually starts in the late autumn, peaks in January to February, and can last until late spring.[76] As long as flu season is in effect, vaccination is indicated.

6. "I'm scared of needles."

Fear of needles is an extremely common reason why patients refuse vaccination. The intranasal vaccine is an option for most healthy, nonpregnant patients between the ages of 2 and 49 years.[78] For those patients not eligible for the intranasal version, a reminder that the minor discomfort from the intramuscular injection pales compared with symptoms and potential complications of the influenza virus itself often convinces those who are hesitant to accept vaccination.

7. "I'm worried about the safety of the vaccine."

Patients who are concerned about vaccine safety can be assured that it is closely monitored by the CDC and US Food and Drug Administration, primarily through the Vaccine Adverse Event Recording System. For more than 50 years, hundreds of millions of vaccines have been administered without adverse events. The only true absolute contraindication to the influenza vaccine is a history of life-threatening reaction to eggs or any other vaccine component.[76]

REFERENCES

1. Martin BL, Nelson MR, Hershey JN, et al. Adverse reactions to vaccines. Clin Rev Allergy Immunol 2003;24:263–75.
2. Miller ER, Haber P, Hibbs B, et al. Chapter 21: surveillance for adverse events following immunization. VPD surveillance manual. 4th edition; Atlanta (GA): Centers for Disease Control and Prevention. Manual for the surveillance of vaccine-preventable diseases. Centers for Disease Control and Prevention; 2008.
3. Kroger AT, Atkinson WL, Marcuse EK, et al, Advisory Committee on Immunization Practices Centers for Disease Control and Prevention. General recommendations on immunization: recommendations of the Advisory Committee on Immunization Practices (ACIP). MMWR Morb Mortal Wkly Rep 2006;55:1–48.
4. Rothstein E, Kohl KS, Ball L, et al. Nodule at injection site as an adverse event following immunization: case definition and guidelines for data collection, analysis, and presentation. Vaccine 2004;22(5/6):576–85.
5. James JM, Burks AW, Robertson PK, et al. Safe administration of the measles vaccine to children allergic to eggs. N Engl J Med 1995;332:1262–6.
6. Sakaguchi M, Nakayama T, Inouye T, et al. Anaphylaxis to gelatin in children with systemic immediate-type reactions, including anaphylaxis, to vaccines. J Allergy Clin Immunol 1996;98:1058–61.
7. Ball LK, Ball R, Pratt RD. Review article: an assessment of thimerosal use in childhood vaccines. Pediatrics 2001;107(5):1147–54.
8. Kelso JM, Li JT. Practice Parameter: adverse reactions to vaccines. Ann Allergy Asthma Immunol 2009;103:S1–14.
9. Wood RA, Setse R, Halsey N. Irritant skin test reactions to common vaccines. J Allergy Clin Immunol 2007;120:478–81.
10. Carey AB, Meltzer EO. Diagnosis and "desensitization" in tetanus vaccine hypersensitivity. Ann Allergy 1992;69:336–8.
11. Wood RA, Berger M, Dreskin SC, et al. An algorithm for treatment of patients with hypersensitivity reactions after vaccines. Pediatrics 2008;122:e771–7.
12. Centers for Disease Control and Prevention. Recommendations of the Advisory Committee on Immunization Practices (ACIP): use of vaccines and immune globulins in persons with altered immunocompetence. MMWR Recomm Rep 1993; 42(RR-4):1.
13. Center for Disease Control and Prevention. Update: vaccine side effects, adverse reactions, contraindications, and precautions: recommendations of the Advisory Committee on Immunization Practices (ACIP). MMWR Morb Mortal Wkly Rep 1996;45:1–35.
14. Centers for Disease Control and Prevention. Guidelines for vaccinating pregnant women from recommendations of the Advisory Committee on Immunization Practices (ACIP). Atlanta (GA): Centers for Disease Control and Prevention; 2007.

15. CDC. Measles, mumps, and rubella-vaccine use and strategies for elimination of measles, rubella, and congenital rubella syndrome and control of mumps: recommendations of the Advisory Committee on Immunization Practices (ACIP). MMWR Recomm Rep 1998;47(RR-8):1–57.
16. CDC. Prevention of varicella: recommendations of the Advisory Committee on Immunization Practices (ACIP). MMWR Recomm Rep 2007;56(RR-4):1–40.
17. CDC. Update: recommendations from the Advisory Committee on Immunization Practices [ACIP] regarding administration of combination MMRV vaccine. MMWR Morb Mortal Wkly Rep 2008;57:258–60.
18. Marin M, Broder KR, Temte JL, et al. Use of combination measles, mumps, rubella, and varicella vaccine: recommendations of the Advisory Committee on Immunization Practices (ACIP). MMWR Recomm Rep 2010;59(RR-3):1–12.
19. Jacobsen SJ, Ackerson BK, Sy LS, et al. Observational safety study of febrile convulsion following first dose MMRV vaccination in a managed care setting. Vaccine 2009;27:4656–61.
20. Sillanpaa M, Camfield P, Camfield C, et al. Incidence of febrile seizures in Finland: prospective population-based study. Pediatr Neurol 2008;38:391–4.
21. Kliegman RM, Berhman RE, Jenson HB, et al. Seizures in childhood. In: Kliegman RM, Berhman RE, Jenson HB, et al, editors. Nelson textbook of pediatrics. 18th edition. Philadelphia: Saunders; 2007. p. 2457–75.
22. Baulac S, Gourfinkel-An I, Nabbout R, et al. Fever, genes, and epilepsy. Lancet Neurol 2004;3:421–30.
23. Barlow WE, Davis RL, Glasser JW, et al. The risk of seizures after receipt of whole-cell pertussis or measles, mumps, and rubella vaccine. N Engl J Med 2001;345:656–61.
24. Vestergaard M, Hviid A, Madsen KM, et al. MMR vaccination and febrile seizures: evaluation of susceptible subgroups and long-term prognosis. JAMA 2004;292:351.
25. Kroger AT, Atkinson WL, Marcuse EK, et al. General recommendations on immunization: recommendations of the Advisory Committee on Immunization Practices. MMWR Recomm Rep 2006;55(RR-15):1–48.
26. Marin M, Güris D, Chaves SC, et al. Prevention of varicella: recommendations of the Advisory Committee on Immunization Practices (ACIP). MMWR Recomm Rep 2007;56(RR04):1–40.
27. Chaves SS, Zhang J, Civen R, et al. Varicella disease in vaccinated persons: clinical and epidemiologic characteristics, 1997–2005. J Infect Dis 2008;197(Suppl 2): S127–31.
28. Kuter B, Matthews H, Shinefield H, et al. Ten year follow-up of healthy children who received one or two injections of varicella vaccine. Pediatr Infect Dis J 2004;23:132–7.
29. Seward JF, Zhang JX, Maupin TJ, et al. Contagiousness of varicella in vaccinated cases: a household contact study. JAMA 2004;292:704–8.
30. Perella D, Fiks A, Spain CV, et al. Validity of reported varicella history as a marker for varicella-zoster virus immunity [Poster]. Presented at: 2005 Pediatric Academic Societies Annual Meeting. Washington, DC, May 14–17, 2005.
31. Bosch FX, De SS. Human papillomavirus and cervical cancer—burden and assessment of causality. J Natl Center Inst Monogr 2003;21:3–13.
32. A human papillomavirus vaccine. Med Lett Drugs Ther 2006;48:65.
33. Myers ER, McCrory DC, Nanda K, et al. Mathematical model for the natural history of human papillomavirus infection and cervical carcinogenesis. Am J Epidemiol 2000;151:1158–71.
34. Manhart LE, Holmes KK, Koutsky LA, et al. Human papillomavirus infection among sexually active young women in the United States: implications for developing a vaccination strategy. Sex Transm Dis 2006;33:502–8.

35. Garland SM, Smith JS. Human papillomavirus vaccines: current status and future prospects. Drugs 2010;70(9):1079–98.
36. Markowitz LE. HPV vaccines–prophylactic, not therapeutic. JAMA 2007;298(7): 805–6.
37. Pagliusi SR, Dillner J, Pawlita M, et al. International standard reagents for harmonization of HPV serology and DNA assays–an update. Vaccine 2006;24: S193–200.
38. Markowitz LE, Dunne EF, Saraiya M, et al. Quadrivalent human papillomavirus vaccine: recommendations of the Advisory Committee on Immunization Practices (ACIP). MMWR Recomm Rep 2007;56:1–23.
39. Cervarix–a second HPV vaccine. Med Lett Drugs Ther 2010;1338:37.
40. Garland SM, Herandez-Avila M, Wheeler CM, et al. Quadrivalent vaccine against human papillomavirus to prevent anogenital diseases. N Engl J Med 2007; 356(19):1928–43.
41. The FUTURE II Study Group. Quadrivalent vaccine against human papillomavirus to prevent high-grade cervical lesions. N Engl J Med 2007;356:1915–27.
42. The FUTURE II Study Group. Prophylactic efficacy of a quadrivalent human papillomavirus (HPV) vaccine in women with virological evidence of HPV infection. J Infect Dis 2007;196(15):1438–46.
43. Mills R, Tyring SK, Levin MJ, et al. Safety, tolerability, and immunogenicity of zoster vaccine in subjects with a history of herpes zoster. Vaccine 2010;28:4204–9.
44. Harpaz R, Ortega-Sanchez IR, Seward JF. Prevention of herpes zoster: recommendations of the Advisory Committee on Immunization Practices (ACIP). MMWR Recomm Rep 2008;57:1.
45. Waregam DW, Breuer J. Herpes zoster. BMJ 2007;334:1211–5.
46. Hornberger J, Robertus K. Cost-effectiveness of a vaccine to prevent herpes zoster and postherpectic neuralgia in older adults. Ann Intern Med 2006;145:317–25.
47. Schmader K. Herpes zoster in older adults. Clin Infect Dis 2001;32(10):1481–6.
48. Herpes zoster vaccine (Zostavax). Med Lett Drugs Ther 2006;48:73.
49. Oxman MN, Levin MJ, Shingles Prevention Study Group. Vaccination against herpes zoster and postherpetic neuralgia. J Infect Dis 2008;197:S228–36.
50. Simberkoff MS, Arbeit RD, Johnson GR, et al. Safety of herpes zoster vaccine in the Shingles Prevention Study: a randomized trial. Ann Intern Med 2010;152(9): 545–54.
51. Advisory Committee on Immunization Practices. Recommended adult immunization schedule: United States, 2010. Ann Intern Med 2010;152:36.
52. Krugman S, Overby LR, Mushahwar IK, et al. Viral hepatitis, type B: studies on natural history and prevention re-examined. N Engl J Med 1979;300:101–6.
53. McMahon BJ, Alward WL, Hall DB, et al. Acute hepatitis B virus infection: relation of age to the clinical expression of disease and subsequent development of the carrier state. J Infect Dis 1985;151:599–603.
54. Dienstag JL. Immunopathogenesis of the extrahepatic manifestations of hepatitis B virus infections. Springer Semin Immunopathol 1981;3:461–72.
55. CDC. Hepatitis surveillance: report number 60. Atlanta (GA): US Department of Health and Human Services, Public Health Service, CDC; 2005.
56. Edmunds WJ, Medley GF, Nokes DJ, et al. The influence of age on the development of the hepatitis B carrier state. Proc Biol Sci 1993;253:197–201.
57. Hyams KC. Risks of chronicity following acute hepatitis B virus infection: a review. Clin Infect Dis 1995;20:992–1000.
58. Hoofnagle JH, DiBisceglie AM. Serologic diagnosis of acute and chronic viral hepatitis. Semin Liver Dis 1991;11:73–83.

59. Alter HJ, Seeff LB, Kaplan PM, et al. Type B hepatitis: the infectivity of blood positive for e antigen and DNA polymerase after accidental needlestick exposure. N Engl J Med 1976;295:909–13.
60. Shikata T, Karasawa T, Abe K, et al. Hepatitis B e antigen and infectivity of hepatitis B virus. J Infect Dis 1977;136:571–6.
61. Alter HJ, Purcell RH, Gerin JL, et al. Transmission of hepatitis B to chimpanzees by hepatitis B surface antigen-positive saliva and semen. Infect Immun 1977;16:928–33.
62. Bancroft WH, Snitbhan R, Scott RM, et al. Transmission of hepatitis B virus to gibbons by exposure to human saliva containing hepatitis B surface antigen. J Infect Dis 1977;135:79–85.
63. Bond WW, Favero MS, Petersen NJ, et al. Survival of hepatitis B virus after drying and storage for one week. Lancet 1981;1(8219):550–1.
64. Mast EE, Margolis HS, Fiore AE. A comprehensive immunization strategy to eliminate transmission of hepatitis B virus infection in the United States. Recommendations of the Advisory Committee on Immunization Practices (ACIP) Part I: immunization of infants, children, and adolescents. MMWR Recomm Rep 2005; 54(RR-16):1–31.
65. Beasley RP, Stevens CE, Shiao IS, et al. Evidence against breast-feeding as a mechanism for vertical transmission of hepatitis B. Lancet 1975;2(7938):740–1.
66. Armstrong GL, Mast EE, Wojczynski M, et al. Childhood hepatitis B virus infections in the United States before hepatitis B immunization. Pediatrics 2001;108:1123–8.
67. Emini EA, Ellis RW, Miller WJ, et al. Production and immunological analysis of recombinant hepatitis B vaccine. J Infect 1986;13(Suppl A):3–9.
68. CDC. Recommended immunization schedule for persons aged 0 through 18—United States, 2011. MMWR 2011;60(5):1–4.
69. McMahon BJ, Dentinger CM, Bruden D, et al. Antibody levels and protection after hepatitis B vaccine: results of a 22-year follow-up study and response to a booster dose. J Infect Dis 2009;200(9):1390–6.
70. U.S. Public Health Service. Updated U.S. Public Health Service Guidelines for the Management of Occupational Exposures to HBV, HCV, and HIV and Recommendations for Postexposure Prophylaxis. MMWR Recomm Rep 2001;50(RR-11):1–42.
71. Hadler SC, Francis DP, Maynard JE, et al. Long-term immunogenicity and efficacy of hepatitis B vaccine in homosexual men. N Engl J Med 1986;315:209–14.
72. CDC. Hepatitis B vaccination coverage among adults–United States, 2004. MMWR Morb Mortal Wkly Rep 2006;55:509–11.
73. Wismans PJ, van Hattum J, de Gast GC, et al. A prospective study of in vitro anti-HBs producing B cells (spot-ELISA) following primary and supplementary vaccination with a recombinant hepatitis B vaccine in insulin dependent diabetic patients and matched controls. J Med Virol 1991;35(3):216–22.
74. Douvin C, Simon D, Charles MA. Hepatitis B vaccination in diabetic patients. Randomized trial comparing recombinant vaccines containing and not containing pre-S2 antigen. Diabetes Care 1997;20(2):148–51.
75. CDC. Recommendations for identification and public health management of persons with chronic hepatitis B virus infection. MMWR Recomm Rep 2008;5(RR-8):1–20.
76. CDC. Prevention and control of influenza and vaccines: recommendations of the Advisory Committee on Immunization Practices (ACIP). MMWR Recomm Rep 2010;59(RR-8):1–62.
77. Thompson WW, Shay DK, Weintraub E, et al. Influenza-associated hospitalization in the United States. JAMA 2004;292(11):1333–40.
78. CDC. Vaccine information statement (interim). Live, Attenuated influenza vaccine (8/10/10) USC §300aa-26.

Index

Note: Page numbers of article titles are in **boldface** type.

Prim Care Clin Office Pract 38 (2011) 777–786
doi:10.1016/S0095-4543(11)00083-2

G

H

Y

Z

United States
Postal Service

Statement of Ownership, Management, and Circulation
(All Periodicals Publications Except Requestor Publications)

1. Publication Title	2. Publication Number	3. Filing Date
Primary Care: Clinics in Office Practice	0 4 4 - 6 9 0	9/16/11
4. Issue Frequency Mar, Jun, Sep, Dec	5. Number of Issues Published Annually 4	6. Annual Subscription Price $203.00

7. Complete Mailing Address of Known Office of Publication (*Not printer*) (*Street, city, county, state, and ZIP+4®*)

Elsevier Inc.
360 Park Avenue South
New York, NY 10010-1710

Contact Person
Stephen Bushing
Telephone (Include area code)
215-239-3688

8. Complete Mailing Address of Headquarters or General Business Office of Publisher (*Not printer*)

Elsevier Inc., 360 Park Avenue South, New York, NY 10010-1710

9. Full Names and Complete Mailing Addresses of Publisher, Editor, and Managing Editor (*Do not leave blank*)

Publisher (*Name and complete mailing address*)

Kim Murphy, Elsevier, Inc., 1600 John F. Kennedy Blvd. Suite 1800, Philadelphia, PA 19103-2899

Editor (*Name and complete mailing address*)

Yonah Korngold, Elsevier, Inc., 1600 John F. Kennedy Blvd. Suite 1800, Philadelphia, PA 19103-2899

Managing Editor (*Name and complete mailing address*)

Barton Dudlick, Elsevier, Inc., 1600 John F. Kennedy Blvd. Suite 1800, Philadelphia, PA 19103-2899

10. Owner (*Do not leave blank. If the publication is owned by a corporation, give the name and address of the corporation immediately followed by the names and addresses of all stockholders owning or holding 1 percent or more of the total amount of stock. If not owned by a corporation, give the names and addresses of the individual owners. If owned by a partnership or other unincorporated firm, give its name and address as well as those of each individual owner. If the publication is published by a nonprofit organization, give its name and address.*)

Full Name	Complete Mailing Address
Wholly owned subsidiary of	4520 East-West Highway
Reed/Elsevier, US holdings	Bethesda, MD 20814

11. Known Bondholders, Mortgagees, and Other Security Holders Owning or Holding 1 Percent or More of Total Amount of Bonds, Mortgages, or Other Securities. If none, check box → ☐ None

Full Name	Complete Mailing Address
N/A	

12. Tax Status (*For completion by nonprofit organizations authorized to mail at nonprofit rates*) (*Check one*)
The purpose, function, and nonprofit status of this organization and the exempt status for federal income tax purposes:
☐ Has Not Changed During Preceding 12 Months
☐ Has Changed During Preceding 12 Months (*Publisher must submit explanation of change with this statement*)

PS Form **3526**, September 2007 (Page 1 of 3 (Instructions Page 3)) PSN 7530-01-000-9931 **PRIVACY NOTICE**: See our Privacy policy in www.usps.com

13. Publication Title: Primary Care: Clinics in Office Practice
14. Issue Date for Circulation Data Below: September 2011

15. Extent and Nature of Circulation		Average No. Copies Each Issue During Preceding 12 Months	No. Copies of Single Issue Published Nearest to Filing Date
a. Total Number of Copies (*Net press run*)		623	426
b. Paid Circulation (By Mail and Outside the Mail)	(1) Mailed Outside-County Paid Subscriptions Stated on PS Form 3541. (*Include paid distribution above nominal rate, advertiser's proof copies, and exchange copies*)	255	235
	(2) Mailed In-County Paid Subscriptions Stated on PS Form 3541 (*Include paid distribution above nominal rate, advertiser's proof copies, and exchange copies*)		
	(3) Paid Distribution Outside the Mails Including Sales Through Dealers and Carriers, Street Vendors, Counter Sales, and Other Paid Distribution Outside USPS®	44	46
	(4) Paid Distribution by Other Classes Mailed Through the USPS (e.g. First-Class Mail®)		
c. Total Paid Distribution (*Sum of 15b (1), (2), (3), and (4)*) ►		299	281
d. Free or Nominal Rate Distribution (By Mail and Outside the Mail)	(1) Free or Nominal Rate Outside-County Copies Included on PS Form 3541	56	54
	(2) Free or Nominal Rate In-County Copies Included on PS Form 3541		
	(3) Free or Nominal Rate Copies Mailed at Other Classes Through the USPS (e.g. First-Class Mail)		
	(4) Free or Nominal Rate Distribution Outside the Mail (Carriers or other means)		
e. Total Free or Nominal Rate Distribution (Sum of 15d (1), (2), (3) and (4))		56	54
f. Total Distribution (Sum of 15c and 15e) ►		355	335
g. Copies not Distributed (See instructions to publishers #4 (page #3)) ►		268	91
h. Total (Sum of 15f and g)		623	426
i. Percent Paid (15c divided by 15f times 100) ►		84.23%	83.88%

16. Publication of Statement of Ownership

☐ If the publication is a general publication, publication of this statement is required. Will be printed in the **December 2011** issue of this publication. ☐ Publication not required

17. Signature and Title of Editor, Publisher, Business Manager, or Owner

Stephen R. Bushing –Inventory Distribution Coordinator

Date: September 16, 2011

I certify that all information furnished on this form is true and complete. I understand that anyone who furnishes false or misleading information on this form or who omits material or information requested on the form may be subject to criminal sanctions (including fines and imprisonment) and/or civil sanctions (including civil penalties).

PS Form 3526, September 2007 (Page 2 of 3)

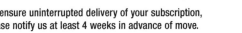

Printed and bound by CPI Group (UK) Ltd, Croydon, CR0 4YY
03/10/2024
01040441-0002